Medical Anthropology

Understanding Public Health

Series editors: Nick Black and Rosalind Raine, London School of Hygiene & Tropical Medicine

Throughout the world, recognition of the importance of public health to sustainable, safe and healthy societies is growing. The achievements of public health in nineteenth-century Europe were for much of the twentieth century overshadowed by advances in personal care, in particular in hospital care. Now, with the dawning of a new century, there is increasing understanding of the inevitable limits of individual health care and of the need to complement such services with effective public health strategies. Major improvements in people's health will come from controlling communicable diseases, eradicating environmental hazards, improving people's diets and enhancing the availability and quality of effective health care. To achieve this, every country needs a cadre of knowledgeable public health practitioners with social, political and organizational skills to lead and bring about changes at international, national and local levels.

This is one of a series of 20 books that provides a foundation for those wishing to join in and contribute to the twenty-first-century regeneration of public health, helping to put the concerns and perspectives of public health at the heart of policy-making and service provision. While each book stands alone, together they provide a comprehensive account of the three main aims of public health: protecting the public from environmental hazards, improving the health of the public and ensuring high quality health services are available to all. Some of the books focus on methods, others on key topics. They have been written by staff at the London School of Hygiene & Tropical Medicine with considerable experience of teaching public health to students from low, middle and high income countries. Much of the material has been developed and tested with postgraduate students both in face-to-face teaching and through distance learning.

The books are designed for self-directed learning. Each chapter has explicit learning objectives, key terms are highlighted and the text contains many activities to enable the reader to test their own understanding of the ideas and material covered. Written in a clear and accessible style, the series will be essential reading for students taking postgraduate courses in public health and will also be of interest to public health practitioners and policy-makers.

Titles in the series

Analytical models for decision making: Colin Sanderson and Reinhold Gruen
Controlling communicable disease: Norman Noah
Economic analysis for management and policy: Stephen Jan, Lilani Kumaranayake, Jenny Roberts, Kara Hanson and Kate Archibald
Economic evaluation: Julia Fox-Rushby and John Cairns (eds)
Environmental epidemiology: Paul Wilkinson (ed)
Environment, health and sustainable development: Megan Landon
Environmental health policy: David Ball
Financial management in health services: Reinhold Gruen and Anne Howarth
Global change and health: Kelley Lee and Jeff Collin (eds)
Health care evaluation: Sarah Smith, Don Sinclair, Rosalind Raine and Barnaby Reeves
Health promotion practice: Maggie Davies, Wendy Macdowall and Chris Bonell (eds)
Health promotion theory: Maggie Davies and Wendy Macdowall (eds)
Introduction to epidemiology: Lucianne Bailey, Katerina Vardulaki, Julia Langham and Daniel Chandramohan
Introduction to health economics: David Wonderling, Reinhold Gruen and Nick Black
Issues in public health: Joceline Pomerleau and Martin McKee (eds)
Making health policy: Kent Buse, Nicholas Mays and Gill Walt
Managing health services: Nick Goodwin, Reinhold Gruen and Valerie Iles
Medical anthropology: Robert Pool and Wenzel Geissler
Principles of social research: Judith Green and John Browne (eds)
Understanding health services: Nick Black and Reinhold Gruen

Medical Anthropology

Robert Pool and Wenzel Geissler

Open University Press

Open University Press
McGraw-Hill Education
McGraw-Hill House
Shoppenhangers Road
Maidenhead
Berkshire
England
SL6 2QL

email: enquiries@openup.co.uk
world wide web: www.openup.co.uk

and Two Penn Plaza, New York, NY 10121-2289, USA

First published 2005

A catalogue record of this book is available from the British Library

ISBN-10: 0 335 21850 4 (pb)
ISBN-13: 978 0 335 21850 9 (pb)

Library of Congress Cataloging-in-Publication Data
CIP data has been applied for

Typeset by RefineCatch Limited, Bungay, Suffolk
Printed in Poland by OZGraf. S.A.
www.polskabook.pl

Contents

Acknowledgements

Open University Press and the London School of Hygiene and Tropical Medicine have made every effort to obtain permission from copyright holders to reproduce material in this book and to acknowledge these sources correctly. Any omissions brought to our attention will be remedied in future editions.

We would like to express our grateful thanks to the following copyright holders for granting permission to reproduce material in this book.

p. 77–86   Amarasingham Rhodes, Lorna, 'Studying biomedicine as a cultural system' in Carolyn F Sargent and Thomas M Johnson (eds), *Medical Anthropology: Contemporary Theory and Method.* Copyright © 1996 by Prager. Reproduced with permission from Greenwood Publishing Group, Inc., Westport, CT.

p. 66–9   Medical Anthropology Quarterly. Online by Michael Bloor, et al. Copyright 1993 by AM ANTHROPOLOGY ASSN (J). Reproduced with permission of AM ANTHROPOLOGY ASSN (J) in the format Textbook via Copyright Clearance Center.

p. 148   Fabian J, *Remembering the Present: Painting and Popular History in Zaire,* by University of California Press. Copyright © 1996 Johannes Fabian. Reproduced with permission from Johannes Fabian.

p. 32–7   Skelton JA and Croyle RT (eds), *Mental Representation in Health and Illness.* Copyright © 1991 Springer-Verlag. Reprinted with permission from Springer-Verlag.

p. 70–4   Farmer P, 'Ethnography, social analysis, and the prevention' in Inhom C and Brown PJ (editors), *The Anthropology of Infectious Diseases,* 1997, Taylor and Francis Books Ltd.

p. 25–6   Geertz C, *The Interpretation of Culture.* Copyright © 1973 by Basic Books. Reprinted by permission of Basic Books, a member of Perseus, L.L.C., and HarperCollins Publishers Ltd.

p. 157–60   First published in *AFRICA,* Journal of the International African Institute, London 2005 and published by kind permission of the IAI.

p. 45–50   Hausmann-Muela S, Ribera JM and Tanner M, 'Fake Malaria and hidden parasites – the ambiguity of Malaria', *Anthropology and Medicine* 5 pp43–61 (2000). © Taylor & Francis Ltd. Journals website: http://www.tandf.co.uk/journals

p. 13   Holston J, *The Modernist City: An Anthropological Critique of Brasilia.* © 1989 by The University of Chicago. All rights reserved.

p. 146   Hoppe KA, 'Lord of the fly: Colonial visions and revisions of African Sleeping Sickness environments on Lake Victoria 1906–1961', *Africa* 67(1), Edinburgh University Press and International African Institute, 1997. Website: www.eup.ed.ac.uk

p. 8–11   Keesing RM and Strathern AJ, *Cultural Anthropology, A Contemporary*

	Perspective 3rd edition. © 1998. Reprinted with permission of Wadsworth, a division of Thomson Learning. www.thomsonrights. com. Fax 800 730–2215.
p. 154	Reprinted from East African Standard. Copyright © Paul Kelemba.
p. 91–7	Nichter M and Nichter M, *Anthropology and International Health: Asian Case Studies*, 1996, Taylor and Francis Books (Gordon Breach).
p. 131–8	American Ethnologist. ONLINE by ONG, A. Copyright 1988 by AM ANTHROPOLOGICAL ASSN (J). Reproduced with permission of AM ANTHROPOLOGICAL ASSN (J) in the format Textbook via Copyright Clearance Center.
p. 17–22, 55–58	Pool R, *Negotiating a Good Death. Euthanasia in the Netherlands*, pp1–9 and 187–193. Copyright © 2000, Haworth Press, Inc., Binghamton, New York.
p. 121–6, 128	Reprinted from *Social Science and Medicine*, Vol 31, No 9, 1990, pp1023–1028. Taylor: 'Condoms and cosmology: the "fractal" person and sexual risk in Rwanda'. Copyright © 1990. Reprinted with permission from Elsevier.
p. 110–15	Whyte SR, et al, 'Treating AIDS: Dilemmas of unequal access in Uganda', 2004, *SAHARA J*, 1(1): 14–16.
p. 54	Young A, 'The Anthropologies of illness and sickness'. Reprinted with permission from the *Annual Review of Anthropology*, Volume 31 © 1982 by Annual Reviews www.annualreviews.org

Overview of the book

Introduction

Recent decades have seen growing participation by medical anthropologists in medical research and public health, and medical anthropology has become the single largest subdiscipline in anthropology. Nowadays an increasing number of medical research projects (at least once they progress beyond the initial laboratory-based phase) and public health interventions involve medical anthropologists – or closely related social science disciplines – in some capacity. Increasingly, anthropologists and health professionals work hand-in-hand in an interdisciplinary effort to alleviate suffering.

However, true interdisciplinarity between the social sciences and medicine remains a challenge for a number of reasons. First, anthropology and biomedicine are based on different assumptions about fundamental issues such as the nature of social reality and how it should be studied. Second, medical research and public health are dominated by biomedicine, and biomedical professionals often have a poor understanding of what anthropology is and what it has to offer (beyond the rapid use of qualitative methods). Third, anthropologists have often failed to communicate with medical professionals and make a convincing case for what anthropology has to offer. Consequently, there is often a need to mediate between people working towards the same goal from different disciplinary perspectives. Apart from respect, mutual understanding of the assumptions and approaches of the other discipline is essential for interdisciplinary co-operation.

This book aims to provide those working in medical research and public health with a basic understanding of some of the anthropological approaches and tools that are relevant to the study of health and illness and to the improvement of the impact and sustainability of health work. It is aimed at those new to anthropology and can thus be used as an introduction to the subdiscipline both for health professionals and for novice social scientists.

Structure of the book

As we see it, medical anthropology is not structured by biomedical categories such as 'mental illness' or 'AIDS' or 'infectious diseases', but by a particular approach. In illustrating what we see as the important elements of this approach we have focused on some of the topic areas relevant to biomedicine, ignoring others. This choice of topics has also been influenced by our own experience and, as a result, the book is coloured by the geographical and thematic interests of its authors.

In the first two chapters we introduce anthropology and discuss its most important characteristics. In Chapter 1 we focus mainly on the anthropological concept of culture. Then, in Chapter 2, we explore the ways in which anthropology approaches the study of culture and society and the perspectives it uses to understand social and cultural phenomena.

In Chapter 3 we introduce the subdiscipline of medical anthropology, and in Chapter 4 we discuss medical systems, often considered to be the main object of medical anthropology. Chapter 5 goes on to examine a number of other concepts that medical anthropologists have developed in their attempts to grapple with the complexity of people's experience of health and sickness: the distinction between illness and disease, illness narratives, and explanatory models.

Chapter 6 looks in more detail at the wider context of sickness and focuses on one particular sickness: HIV/AIDS.

Chapter 7 examines the relationship between anthropology and biomedicine in more detail and discusses some of the ways in which interdisciplinary collaboration could be developed.

In Chapter 8, we move on to medicines and explore some social and cultural factors that influence their use and efficacy. As objectifications of medical knowledge, medicines can move between very different contexts. In Chapter 9, this is illustrated by the case of Western pharmaceutical companies.

Chapter 10 turns to another area of anthropology that is critical to medicine and public health: the study of different notions of what a person is, and different moralities of what people should be, which influence the body, health and treatment. Notions of personhood and relatedness, which social anthropology studies, shape ideas and practices around the body and thus health-seeking practices, but these notions are themselves not stable in a radically changing world; thus conflicts between social groups and whole societies can be played out through illnesses of individuals, which we explore here by looking at cases of spirit possession.

Finally, we look at how anthropology can help us to understand ourselves better by studying medical research and public health interventions as socially productive networks. Chapter 11 includes some historical dimensions into medical anthropology, and in Chapter 12 we suggest that we ought to begin medical anthropological studies by looking at ourselves, researchers and implementers in public health, making research projects or the health interventions into objects of anthropological research. This reflexive ending applies the concepts of ethnography and participant observation, developed in the first chapters, to public health workers, that is to the readers themselves.

The book thus takes us from one set of concerns of medical anthropology – understanding often very different medicinal practices – to another one: understanding ourselves and our own medicinal ideas and practices. Our aim is to show that these two concerns cannot be separated and should be linked in an anthropological approach.

As we move through these different subject areas, we draw on our own personal research and experiences, as well as abridged literature by other authors to illustrate important concepts, approaches and insights. If you are particularly interested in the topic, we have included references to the original texts. The aim of reading these texts, apart from understanding the argument, is to find your own position –

do you agree or not, and why? – and to identify links between the texts and your own experience. The references at the end of each chapter provide details of further optional reading.

Each chapter includes:

- an overview
- a list of learning objectives
- a list of key terms
- a range of activities
- feedback on the activities
- a summary

After the reading tasks you will find questions and some brief feedback to the questions. This feedback should not be seen as an alternative to a careful reading of the texts.

It is our hope that the range of materials and cases will convey some of the interest of medical anthropology.

Acknowledgement

The authors would like to acknowledge the contribution of Professor Sheila Hiller, Queen Mary, University of London, for reviewing this book, and Deirdre Byrne, series manager for help and support.

Anthropology and culture

Overview

In this chapter and the next we will introduce anthropology and discuss its most important characteristics. First we define anthropology and discuss the central concept of culture. Then, in the next chapter, we present other key aspects such as participant observation, comparison and holism.

Learning objectives

By the end of this chapter you should be able to:

- **define anthropology**
- **describe the main mistaken assumptions on which health professionals base their interest in anthropology**
- **explain the anthropological concept of culture**

Key terms

Epistemology A branch of philosophy concerned with the nature of knowledge, the different kinds of knowledge that are possible and their limits.

Ethnocentrism The assumption that your own culture, values, ways of doing things – the ones that you have learned and internalized – are the only or the best or the most valid ones.

Heuristic Allowing or assisting to discover. In social science, a heuristic device is a model or a concept that, while not necessarily portraying things as they really are, nonetheless helps us to understand them (for example, 'culture' or 'medical system').

Reification When an abstraction that we have created to help us to understand reality (for example, a concept or a model) is seen as something concrete, which really exists and exerts a causal influence (for example, culture causes risk behaviour).

What is anthropology?

Anthropology. 1. the study of mankind, esp. of its societies and customs. 2. the study of the structure and evolution of man as an animal. (*Oxford English Dictionary*)

The word 'anthropology' (from the Greek *anthropos* = humankind, *logos* = discourse) means the study of people in its broadest sense. It includes physical or biological anthropology, involving the study of human evolution, and sociocultural anthropology that, very generally speaking, entails studying the social and cultural aspects of human society. In this book, when we use the term 'anthropology' we will be referring to sociocultural anthropology.

Sociocultural anthropology is, in turn, divided into a number of subspecializations: political anthropology (studying political processes and the exercise of power in different settings), economic anthropology (studying exchange and other economic phenomena from a sociocultural perspective), the anthropology of religion (focusing on religion as a sociocultural practice and experience), the anthropology of kinship (studying social relations, especially within the family, and how these are culturally produced), and medical anthropology (which studies the social and cultural aspects of health and illness). There are many more subspecializations. This chapter and the next will describe the main characteristics of sociocultural anthropology. Chapter 3 will introduce the subdiscipline of medical anthropology.

Anthropology is not a monolithic discipline. In fact, it is tempting to say that there are many different anthropologies. Anthropology occupies the uneasy space between the sciences and the humanities, and it is possible to find individual anthropologists and groupings of anthropologists at almost any position between these two poles.

Many anthropologsts follow Clifford Geertz in insisting that anthropology is 'not an experimental science in search of law but an interpretive one in search of meaning' (Geertz 1973); that it is more like literature than science, and that the interpretation of culture is more like understanding a poem or a novel than explaining the laws of behaviour. There are anthropologists who publish their findings as scientific treatises, and there are anthropologists who publish their findings as poetry.

These differences are not trivial and they have consequences for any attempt to apply anthropology practically, for example in public health. They are grounded in fundamental *epistemological* questions: What are the limits of what we can know about human society? How reliable is this knowledge? Do the things we know about exist separately and independently of our knowledge of them? What kind of knowledge should anthropology seek, and what kind of knowledge can it attain? Is this fundamentally different from, say, medical knowledge?

Public health and anthropology

During the last few decades medical researchers and public health specialists have shown an increasing interest in anthropology. The main reason for this interest has been the realization that there is more to health and disease than physical and biological processes. It has become clear that in order to overcome barriers to the uptake of health interventions and develop culturally appropriate, sustainable interventions, it is first necessary to understand the social and cultural context of health and disease. Much of the enthusiasm for including anthropology in medical research has been based on the assumption that anthropology holds the key to target populations' 'culture' – that is, their beliefs, attitudes and practices (and in particular the supposedly wrong beliefs, misconceptions and risk behaviours that contribute to ill health) – and that anthropologists can advise on how to improve adherence in clinical trials or influence and change problematic beliefs, attitudes and behaviours through culturally appropriate interventions.

There are two things wrong with this approach:

1 The approach is based on wrong assumptions about the nature of anthropology and what it has to offer to public health. It tends to define anthropology in methodological terms, as a set of procedures (qualitative methods, in-depth interviews, focus group discussions) for collecting hidden or sensitive data, for discovering 'cultural' barriers to change, or for discovering 'culturally appropriate' categories for use in survey design.
2 It is also based on wrong assumptions about the nature of society and social processes; namely it assumes that they are determinate, that they are explainable in terms of relatively straightforward causal relationships, and that they can be manipulated and engineered in a preplanned manner with anticipated outcomes.

In the mid-1990s surveillance had shown that there was a relatively high prevalence of HIV in the fishing villages along the shores of Lake Victoria in Tanzania. A development organization requested some anthropological research in these villages to find out what social and cultural factors were contributing to high-risk behaviour (sexual promiscuity). A project supervisor suggested that a team of local researchers should spend two weeks in the villages doing some focus group discussions and in-depth interviews, and then report back on the underlying reasons for this behaviour (i.e. people's beliefs and attitudes). It did not seem to occur to anyone that this would produce a simplified and probably grossly inaccurate picture of what was really happening in these very diverse and complex communities. This would be akin to sending a Tanzanian anthropologist into, say, the red light district in Amsterdam, with the instruction to report on the local 'beliefs and practices' two weeks later. Instead, a longer and more detailed study was suggested. The supervisor was shocked. 'But there is an epidemic and people are dying', she said. 'We can't wait that long. We need results *now* so we can set up interventions.' That was in 1993. Ten years later, after many rapid and applied 'anthropological' studies, they were not really any closer to understanding what was happening in those fishing villages.

Because culture is at the heart of anthropology, and because this is one of the main reasons that health professionals are interested in anthropology, we will first focus, in what follows, on the anthropological concept of culture. You will then learn about the simplified, social engineering approach to society and social change that tends to underlie many public health interventions.

The anthropological concept of culture

Culture. 1. The arts and other manifestations of human intellectual achievement regarded collectively (e.g. Paris as a centre of culture). 2. The customs, civilisation and achievements of a particular time or people (e.g. Chinese culture). 3. Improvement by physical or mental training. (*Oxford English Dictionary*)

Activity 1.1

Read the abridged extract on the anthropological concept of culture, taken from the book *Cultural Anthropology. A Contemporary Perspective*, by Roger Keesing and Andrew Strathern (1998).

As you read it, consider:

1 What is the ideational concept of culture?
2 What problems are associated with viewing others in terms of our own (unconscious) cultural assumptions and values?
3 Where is culture situated: is it a psychological phenomenon in the minds of individuals, or is it a social one situated in the interactions between people?

Anthropological views of culture

The anthropological concept of culture has been one of the most important and influential ideas in twentieth-century thought. Usage of the term *culture* adopted by nineteenth-century anthropologists has spread to other fields of thought with profound impact; it is now commonplace to speak, say, of 'Japanese culture.'

An ideational concept of culture

We will use the term sociocultural system to refer to the pattern of residence, resource exploitation, and so on, characteristic of people. We will restrict the term *culture* to an ideational system: systems of shared ideas, systems of concepts and rules and meanings that underlie and are expressed in the ways that humans live. Culture, so defined, refers to what humans *learn*, not what they do and make.

Perceiving cultural codes

An initial difficulty in the study of culture is that we are not in the habit of analysing cultural patterns; we seldom are even aware of them. It is as though we grow up perceiving the world through glasses with distorting lenses. The things, events, and relationships we assume to be 'out there' are in fact filtered. The first reaction, inevitably, on encountering people who wear a different kind of glasses is to dismiss their behaviour as strange or wrong. To view other ways of life in terms of our own cultural glasses is called *ethnocentrism*. Becoming conscious of, and analytic about, our own cultural glasses is a painful business. We do so best by learning about other people's glasses. Although we can never take our glasses off to find out what the world is 'really like,' or try looking through anyone else's without ours on as well, we can at least learn a good deal out our own prescription.

With some mental effort we can begin to become conscious of the codes that normally lie hidden beneath our everyday behaviour. Consider the mental operations you perform when you go into an unfamiliar supermarket with a shopping list. You have a generalized mental guide to the sections a supermarket will have: one with fresh fruits and vegetables, one with bread, one with fresh meats, one with ice creams and frozen desserts, and so on. In all this, you are drawing on a vastly intricate system of knowledge that is stored in your brain but is only partly accessible to our consciousness. The knowledge in your mental guidebook is not quite like that of other shoppers. But your knowledge and theirs are sufficiently similar that you avoid bumping into one another most of the time, and you avoid violating implicit codes of physical intimacy, eye contact, and orientation in space – as well as eventually finding the groceries you are looking for. Project from the supermarket to the vast body of other shared understandings we need in order to eat in a restaurant, drive in traffic, dress so as to convey the desired impression, or play a game of tennis – and what the anthropologist means by culture will begin to come into view.

We are not, in our everyday lives, simply choosing appropriate alternatives for acting; we are interpreting one another, placing constructions on one another's actions and meanings. Cashing a check at the bank or going to the doctor's office is not simply an enactment of culturally 'programmed' routines, but a *social* process in which the bank teller and customer, or doctor and patient, communicate in ways that require shared understandings. In many settings the capacities in which we relate to one another are less clear-cut, so that social interaction entails negotiating and defining relationships with one another (not simply enacting appropriate roles). Is a lecturer met off campus to be related to by a student formally or informally, as teacher or as acquaintance? How are people who were once lovers to relate to one another? The clues and cues and understandings are at once cultural and individual matters of shared (though unconscious) convention and personal style.

Cultures as systems of shared meanings

Culture consists of shared ideas and meanings. Clifford Geertz, borrowing from the philosopher Gilbert Ryle, provides an interesting example. Consider a wink and an involuntary eye twitch. As physical events, they may be identical – measuring them will not distinguish the two. One is a signal, in a code of meanings Americans share (but which presumably would be unintelligible to Inuits or Australian Aborigines); the other is not. Only in a universe of shared meaning do physical sounds and events become intelligible and convey information.

An anthropological parable – one that happens to be true – will usefully illustrate the nature of cultural meanings. A Bulgarian woman was serving dinner to a group of her American husband's friends, including an Asian student. After her guests had cleaned their plates, she asked if any would like a second helping – a Bulgarian hostess who let a guest go hungry would be disgraced. The Asian student accepted a second helping, and then a third, as the hostess anxiously prepared another batch in the kitchen. Finally, in the midst of his fourth helping, the Asian student slumped to the floor; but better that, in his country, than to insult his hostess by refusing food that had been offered. A Bulgarian hostess serving a second or third helping is not part of Bulgarian culture; but the conceptual principles that lie behind her acts, the patterns of meaning that make them intelligible, are. Bulgarian culture is something learned, something in the minds of Bulgarians, and thus it cannot be studied or observed directly. Nor could our Bulgarian woman tell us all the premises and principles on which her behaviour is based. Many are as hidden from her perception as they are from ours.

When we say that Bulgarian culture is an ideational system, that it is manifest in the minds of Bulgarians, we raise a thorny philosophical issue. Does that mean that a culture is ultimately a psychological system that exists in individual minds? Is Bulgarian culture 'in the heads' of individual Bulgarians?

Geertz's position is that cultural meanings are *public*, and transcend their realization in individual minds. A Beethoven quartet exists in a sense that transcends individuals knowing it, performing it, or printing the score.

Culture as public, culture as private

Those who, like Geertz, argue that cultures are systems of public meanings, not private codes in the minds of individual members, point to the way 'Bulgarian culture' exists prior to (and irrespective of) the birth of any individual Bulgarian. They point to the way that – like the Bulgarian language – it consists of rules and meanings that transcend individual minds. They argue that as a conceptual system, Bulgarian culture is structured in (and changes in) ways that cannot be grasped if we take it to be a composite of what individual Bulgarians know.

Here we get to the heart of the problem. In real communities, the knowledge of the world organized in the minds of individuals varies from person to person, from subgroup to subgroup, from region to region, and varies according to age and sex and life experience and perspective. Yet individuals share a common code, mainly submerged beneath consciousness, that enables them to communicate, to live and work in groups, to anticipate and interpret one another's behaviour. They share a world of common meanings: even though the vantage points individuals have on it are different. In describing 'a culture,' anthropologists are trying to capture what is shared, the code of shared 'rules' and common meanings. We describe a cultural system or a culture when our focus is on the common elements of the code in the community (just as linguists speak of 'the English language,' rather than a local dialect or individual variations).

Moreover, the organization of individuals' knowledge of the world, like the organization of language, is limited and shaped by the structures of mind and brain. A community's heritage of cultural knowledge is subject to many 'real world' constraints: it must lead people to reproduce, raise children, provide food, and organize their social life in ways that sustain the population within an ecosystem, or it will not survive as a cultural tradition. But a cultural tradition, as a composite of individuals' conceptualisations of their world, must also (like a language) be learnable and usable.

The dangers of reification

'A culture' is always a composite, an *abstraction* created as an analytical simplification. We make such a simplification in order to capture and describe as a system the shared elements of socially distributed knowledge. But there is a danger of taking this abstraction we have created as having a concreteness, an existence as an entity and causal agent 'it' cannot have. Both specialists and nonspecialists are prone to talk about 'a culture' as if it could be a causative agent ('their culture leads them to go on vision quests') or a conscious being ('X culture values individuality'). They are prone to talk as if 'a culture' could *do* things ('their culture has adapted to a harsh environment') or to talk as if 'a culture' were, like a group, something one could 'belong to' ('a member of another culture'). We need to guard against the temptation to reify and falsely concretise culture as a 'thing,' to remember that 'it' is a strategically useful abstraction from the distributed knowledge of individuals in communities.

Cultural meanings as social process

Although culture refers to knowledge distributed among individuals in communities, the sharing of meanings in people's daily lives is a social process, not a private me.

Here again we have to force ourselves to think about familiar experiences in unfamiliar ways. If we imagine a community of individuals, each with his or her private conceptualisation of the social world, and each enacting routines and interpreting meanings on the basis of this private conceptualisation of reality, we fail to grasp the social process whereby shared meanings are created and sustained – a process which happens, as it were, *between* people, not simply in their private thought worlds.

The most compelling reasons to interpret social action in terms of ideational codes, not simply to analyse the stream of behaviour, come from the study of language. Much of what we perceive in the world and cloak with meaning is not in the physical world at all. We put it there in our 'mind's eye.' Nevertheless, it is a synthesis of the experiences of individuals and populations encoded over time.

Feedback

1 The ideational concept of culture entails seeing cultures as sets of ideas that we learn and internalize through shared practice. On an unconscious level culture influences much of what we do and how we do it, but we are often not aware of this. It is like distorting glasses that we don't see ourselves but through which we observe the world around us. You should bear in mind that the concept of culture is a heuristic device. It helps us to think about and better understand what people do and why they do it; it does not exist as a 'thing' that independently causes behaviour.

2 Viewing other ways of life uncritically in terms of our own cultural perspectives is called *ethnocentrism*, which leads to bias, intolerance and discrimination. It can be avoided by becoming aware of our own cultural biases through studying and interacting with people whose culture differs from ours (we will discuss the importance of difference and comparison in anthropology in the next chapter).

3 Culture is both in people's heads and social. Keesing and Strathern use the analogy of language to explain this. A language can only exist because individual speakers know it, but individual speakers may know bits that others do not know and so the language as a collective phenomenon is always more than any individual knows of it. Although groups of people share a common code and common meanings, there are also regional, local and individual differences. When we talk about a culture, we are referring to the commonalities, just as when we speak of the English language we are referring to what people who speak English have in common rather than to dialects and individual variations. Meaning (whether linguistic or cultural) is based on individual people's knowledge of the code or the rules, but it is generated in the interaction between individuals, and it exceeds the sum of the individual contributions.

Activity 1.2

Think of an example from your own experience in which hitherto unconscious assumptions or ways of doing things suddenly appeared to you as culturally situated.

⟳ **Feedback**

Your answer will of course depend on your own experience. Here is a simple example
to illustrate this. Having spent many years living in Holland, one of the authors (Robert
Pool) became used to shaking hands when meeting or being introduced to someone.
On arriving in a village in Cameroon, he was surprised to find that some men eagerly
reciprocated when he put out his hand, whereas others either held their hands stiffly
behind their backs or, after an uncomfortable pause, reluctantly extended a flaccid hand,
which was quickly withdrawn after the briefest of contacts. These incidents led to his
discovery of an elaborate set of rules (applied unconsciously as second nature by
everyone else in the village) relating to who could and could not be touched.

Later, living in England, he discovered that hand shaking is much more restricted than in
continental Europe, and that touching people is generally more restricted than in many
other countries.

Social processes and praxis

At the beginning of this chapter we stated that much medical and public health
interest in anthropology is based on the assumption that social processes are
determinate and can be manipulated and in a preplanned manner, with anticipated outcomes. One of the main reasons for wanting to know about people's
beliefs, attitudes and practices, and in particular their wrong beliefs and misconceptions – in other words, their 'culture' – is so that these can be influenced and
rectified through interventions. However, we might question whether it is possible
(and desirable) to change social practices and processes in a preordained and
scientific manner.

In his book *Seeing Like a State: How Certain Schemes to Improve the Human Condition
Have Failed* (1998), the anthropologist James C. Scott examines a number of
large state-sponsored social engineering schemes to understand why they failed.
Focusing on the Soviet collectivization of agriculture, the Tanzanian and Ethiopian
socialist villages, and the building of the cities of Brasilia and Chandigar, Scott
wants to understand why these projects failed. He identifies a number of elements
that underlie such schemes. Here we will focus on two of these that have most
relevance for public health: transformative state simplification and high-modernist
ideology:

- **Transformative state simplification.** According to Scott, various aspects of
  state formation were basically attempts at legibility, simplification, rationaliza-
  tion, for example the invention of permanent last names, freehold land tenure,
  population registers, the standardization of language, and urban planning:
  'In each case, officials took exceptionally complex, illegible, and local social
  practices . . . and created a standard grid whereby it could be centrally recorded
  and monitored.' These simplifications enable greater state control of the population (through taxation and military conscription), but they also enable finely
  tuned interventions (such as public health and poor relief).
- **High-modernist ideology.** This is characterized by confidence about scientific
  and technical progress, the expansion of production, the growing satisfaction of

human needs, the mastery of nature and the rational design of social order. It is
scientifically optimistic – not critical or sceptical. This is often seen in visual
aesthetic terms: a rationally organized city or farm is one that *looks* orderly in a
geometrical sense. See for example the contrast between the 'messy' streets of
Sao Paulo and the 'rational' order of Brasilia.

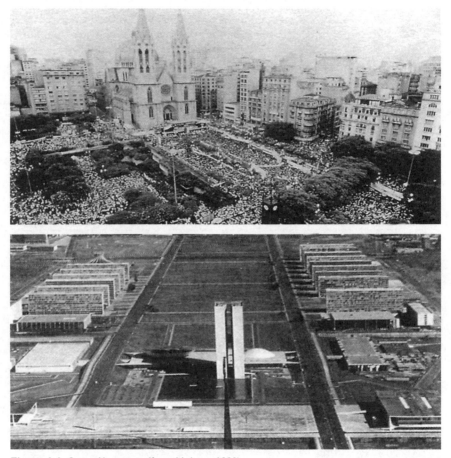

Figure 1.1 *Seeing like a state* (from Holston 1989)

The same visual aesthetic can be found in both the history of public health and in
modern health care (for example, see the discussion of the colonial anti-sleeping
sickness campaigns in early twentieth-century Uganda in Chapter 11).

Reasons for failure

So why did many of these modernist projects fail? For one thing, 'designed or
planned social order ignores essential features of any real, functioning social order'.

Scott illustrates this with the example of the work-to-rule strike, which is based on the fact that any production process (indeed any social process) is based on a whole complex of informal practices and improvisations. By excluding these practices and keeping strictly to the formal rules, workers can halt production. In the same way, Scott argues, because the rules behind the planned city or the collective farm made no allowance for – or even suppressed – informal processes and practices, they were unable to ensure a functioning social order.

Real societies and social processes are too complex, too messy, and too indeterminate to be changed by interventions based exclusively on knowledge of social and cultural 'rules', however accurate. What is missing here is practical knowledge: knowledge embedded in local practice – *praxis*. We will discuss how anthropology studies this praxis in the next chapter.

The point here, of course, is not that there are no social communities in cities like Brasilia, but that communities struggle to exist despite the planners, and the negative social consequences of such planned living arrangements are well known, as are the creative ways in which communities try to overcome the short sightedness of planners. The point of the example is that planned interventions that appear rational and ordered, often do not function as intended.

Summary

Because health and disease are increasingly seen as social as well as biological phenomena, health professionals are becoming interested in anthropology. It is often assumed that because anthropologists study culture (beliefs, attitudes) they are in a good position to advise on how to alter 'misconceptions', improve adherence and influence risk behaviours through culturally appropriate interventions. It is assumed that anthropology consists of qualitative methods that allow relatively easy access to the problematic aspects of people's culture and that once the problem is identified, interventions can be developed to change these. From an anthropological perspective, however, culture is infinitely more complex. It is both individual and social, and can be seen as a set of rules or a code influencing what people do and how they do it. However, it is not enough to 'discover' the underlying social rules of a society or its cultural code. People do not simply enact rules, they improvise and are creative, and in order to understand what people do and why they do it we need to study processes as they are enacted, or praxis. We will come back to this in the next chapter.

References

Geertz C (1973) *The Interpretation of Cultures*. New York: Basic Books.
Hoppe KA (1997) Lords of the fly: colonial visions and revisions of African sleeping sickness environments on Ugandan Lake Victoria. *Africa* 67: 86–105.
Keesing RM and Strathern AJ (1998) *Cultural Anthropology. A Contemporary Perspective*. New York: Holt, Rinehart & Winston.
Scott JC (1998) *Seeing Like a State: How Certain Schemes to Improve the Human Condition Have Failed*. New Haven: Yale University Press.

2 Anthropological perspectives

Overview

In this chapter we explore the ways in which anthropology approaches the study of culture and society and the perspectives it uses to understand social and cultural phenomena. We will also discuss how it presents its findings.

Learning objectives

By the end of this chapter you should understand:

- **the central role of fieldwork in studying how culture is enacted in practical settings**
- **the importance of comparison and difference in this process**
- **the importance of holism, or the inclusion of the wider context of the phenomenon you are studying**
- **why and how anthropologists present their findings as detailed 'thick' descriptions**

Key terms

Cultural relativism The notion that what is good or right or normal in one society is not necessarily so in another.

Ethnography A word with many meanings. 'Ethnography' literally means description of a people or 'ethnic' group. The descriptions that anthropologists write of the people they study are called ethnographies. 'Ethnography' also refers to the actual fieldwork on which anthropologists base their descriptions. Anthropologists *do* ethnography. Sometimes the word is used more broadly to refer to the discipline of anthropology itself.

Positivism The view that there is a reality that exists outside and independently of the observer and that it can be directly apprehended. That the scientific method is the only way of getting accurate information on this reality, and that value judgements and subjective experiences cannot be a valid basis for knowledge.

Presence (participant observation)

Participant observation has always been the main research tool of the anthropologist. It implies that the researcher joins the group that is to be studied –

traditionally another culture – and participates in its activities. The researcher is always around to observe people's actions from close at hand, and having done this for an extended period of time, often several years, he or she is able to develop an understanding of what people are doing and why. The stereotype participant observer is someone who is an insider, who views things through the eyes of the local inhabitants, the insiders, but who is simultaneously an outsider, who notices and critically appraises actions and explanations that are taken for granted by the natives, placing them in a wider context and thus generating understanding.

The extent to which outside anthropologists can 'really' participate in the life of people in another culture has been the subject of much debate. Anthropologists often do not speak the vernacular fluently (especially in the early stages of fieldwork), they often come from a different ethnic, cultural or class background and may lack the cultural competence necessary to interpret what is happening around them properly. And, of course, everyone in the research community knows that the anthropologist is observing them, so they all put on their best behaviour.

These considerations not withstanding, the basic fact of ethnography is that the researcher is *present*, and asking questions. One of the fundamental advantages of being present for extended periods of time, is that relevant and interesting information is more likely to surface in informal contexts than in formal interview settings. This is particularly true of information about topics that are sensitive or hidden – including those that are hidden from the insiders themselves because they have become routinized (see the discussion of culture and practice in Chapter 1). And, to get that information you need to be there.

One of the most important objections to this type of field research is that the data that it produces may be biased. In order to prevent this, it is argued that researchers should try to exclude their own views and preconceptions in order not to 'contaminate' their model of what the people they are studying are doing. Another important objection focuses on the problem of 'informant accuracy' – the fact that different informants may say different things about the same topic.

✐ Activity 2.1

Think about the critique of the social engineering approach in the previous chapter, and especially the concluding discussion of the importance of practical knowledge. On the basis of this, how could you formulate a rebuttal of the objections that participant observation produces biased information?

↻ Feedback

Rather than trying to argue that participant observation can generate unbiased data if the anthropologist can manage to exclude his or her own contaminating influence, you could argue that because practical, situated knowledge is part of all social interaction it might be preferable to recognize this fact and include the knowledge thus gained as part of the anthropologist's data. We will discuss this in some detail below.

Criticisms of bias and contamination are based on untenable assumptions about the nature of social processes, social knowledge, everyday communication, our attempts to study these and our resulting scientific knowledge. Social researchers *always* influence the reality they study: recording conversations, or simply the presence of a researcher or a tape recorder, influences what people say, how they say it and how they act. This also applies to quantitative survey research, although this influence tends to be concealed by the nature of the research procedures and instruments. Social knowledge is always positional, shaped by the observer's point of view, and there is no independent vantage point from which to view, neutrally, a given society. In ethnographic research this positioning is (potentially) more visible. The following experience that one of the authors (Robert Pool) had illustrates this:

> During the early 1990s I carried out a two-year ethnographic study of end-of-life decisions (in particular those relating to euthanasia – which was still illegal at the time) in a hospital in the Netherlands. During the first weeks of participant observation I thought that I would be relatively inconspicuous in my white coat, among the doctors and medical students: I sat next to doctors during consultations and I accompanied them on their rounds; I was there when doctors informed patient of their diagnosis and prognosis, and I was there when doctors discussed treatment options with colleagues. Everyone knew, of course, that I was there and what I was doing, but I assumed that they would soon get used to my presence and not, as far as their decision making was concerned, take any notice of me. Then one day, as I was browsing through a patient's file, I read: 'The patient has expressed the desire for euthanasia. Robert Pool will discuss this with him this afternoon. We await his findings.' I was shocked. I was indeed going to speak to the patient, but certainly not to evaluate his euthanasia request. Doctors started to ask me for my opinion on certain euthanasia requests, and on the odd occasion I was asked to write a report in a patient's case notes. I had become an expert. I was relatively neutral, I was familiar with all those involved, I knew the various points of view and I had an overview of the whole social situation of particular patients. I had plenty of time to discuss at leisure with all those involved and was in a good position to identify misunderstandings and place apparently contradictory statements, actions and interpretations in their wider context. I could not refuse to contribute (and in some cases it would have even been unethical to do so) and as a result I could not avoid influencing what I was studying (Pool 2000).

This influence is not a methodological flaw that must be hidden but an integral aspect of this kind of research that we should accept and make explicit in the presentation of results. Variations in accounts and explanations of the same situation by different respondents (and even by the same respondent at different times) and a degree of indeterminacy, particularly in relation to situations characterized by uncertainty and ambiguity, are an integral part of ethnographic research (because they are part of human social interaction). Informants do not always have ready answers to our questions. Sometimes questions are left unanswered, informants go home and think about them, discuss them and come back with tentative answers that they may have negotiated with others. With these answers they confront our own tentative answers, formed, in the meantime, in discussions with other informants. During fieldwork interpretations constantly change as a result of the anthropologist's conversations with informants but their interpretations are also changing as a result of their conversations with us, and with each other. Surveys do not avoid this, they merely keep it hidden.

A different aspect of this emerges from the study of euthanasia mentioned above. After the completion of fieldwork the major participants met to discuss the book that had been drafted. They tape recorded their discussion and sent it to the anthropologist. A fragment of this discussin shows the influence of the presence of the researcher on their perception of how frequently euthanasia, or euthanasia requests, occurred.

> *Doctor:* What strikes me is that the last year has been so quiet as far as euthanasia goes. When I think about the last case of euthanasia I was involved in, I really have to think back. Whereas when Robert was here I had the feeling that they were coming at me from every corner. If I ran into him and he asked me whether anything had happened I would say: 'You've missed this and you've missed that but perhaps you can still catch this'.

> *Psychologist:* But don't you think that it was his presence that made you realize how often it really occurred? Because there are a lot of situations that never end up as euthanasia, but he was interested in them and enquired about them, and so focused our attention on them. Sometimes he asked me whether anything had happened, and I was convinced that I hadn't forgotten to inform him, but then he would say: 'What about so-and-so?' and then I thought: 'Damn it, you're right'. So it seems like I forget things like that relatively easily and have to be reminded.

> *Doctor:* Yes, now that you mention it, when I think back over the last few months I can recall three cases (Pool 2000: 110).

The anthropologist's presence focused attention on euthanasia so that it seemed to coincide with an increase in its incidence. During the first months in the hospital this was sometimes the subject of jokes, with doctors making remarks like: 'This is the third request this month. Are you sure you're not putting them up to it for your study?' In the discussion it is striking that one of the doctors at first says that there have not been many requests for euthanasia in the last few months, only to realize that there had been at least three. It is worth pondering the implications of this for the reliability of quantitative survey data on the incidence of euthanasia.

Denis Tedlock generalizes the problem thus:

> The more a fieldworker knows and is known, the less that fieldworker can avoid joining the action. The other side of this is that the less a fieldworker knows and is known, the greater will be that fieldworker's inability to interpret the actions of others, whether those actions take him into account or not (Tedlock 1983: 287).

So ethnography is not a process in which objective data are gathered by applying neutral methods, and interviews are not simply a means of information transfer. In this connection the anthropologist Johannes Fabian speaks of *performative* as opposed to *informative* ethnography. Sometimes, he says, the information that the researcher wants is not there, in people's heads, ready to be called up and expressed in discursive statements that can then be collected and taken home as 'data': it has to be made present through enactment, performance.

In fact, once one sees matters in this light, the answers we get to our ethnographic questions can be interpreted as so many cultural performances. Cultural knowledge is always mediated by 'acting'. Performances . . . although they can be asked for, are not really responses to questions. The ethnographer's role, then, is no longer that of questioner; he or she is but a provider of occasions, a catalyst in the weakest sense, and a producer in the strongest (Fabian 1990: 6–7).

Activity 2.2

Go back to Chapter 1 and reread the discussion, in the text by Keesing and Strathern, about meanings as social process. Also remind yourself of the idea of practical knowledge, introduced at the end at the chapter. How do these relate to the discussion above?

Feedback

In society, meaning is created in situations of social interaction between people. In such interaction people do not simply enact rules, beliefs, knowledge; they improvise and are creative, and their knowledge is embedded in this local practice. When anthropologists (or other social scientists, or epidemiologists and medical researchers, for that matter) study this knowledge and these interactions, they become part of the creative process, thus influencing and partly constituting what they are describing.

This obviously does not apply to all knowledge in the same way. Some forms of knowledge, such as *technical knowledge*, are highly systematized and practical activities based on that knowledge are relatively rational and predictable. In interviews with villagers about agricultural techniques, or with doctors about the prognosis and treatment of a common disease, there is not likely to be a lot of uncertainty and negotiation about the right answers. In other domains, less systematic *social knowledge* plays a greater role and actions are determined to a far greater extent by contingent factors such as situation, mood, personality, implicit communication. In such cases it may be difficult for those involved to explain why they acted as they did, or to make the rules governing their actions fully explicit. It is this social knowledge that is often the main focus of anthropology.

Experience

Fieldwork – participant observation – is generally described in textbooks on social science research as a method. But the experience of fieldwork has a much more fundamental role in anthropology: it is what defines anthropology, constitutes its identity, and separates it from other related disciplines like sociology. So what does this experience entail? We illustrate this with another abridged extract from the study of euthanasia (Pool 2000: 1–11).

The end: the death of David

David was one of Dr Edelman's AIDS patients. I had seen him often during more than one and a half year's research in the hospital. He had signed a euthanasia declaration more than six months previously and one day I asked him why he had done so.

'My partner died two years ago,' he said. 'He held out to the very last day. He suffered, I could see he was suffering, and there's no way that I would want to go through *that*. So I think the good part of it is that I can say when. I'm in control'. Dr Edelman's promise to accede to David's euthanasia request in due course was a guarantee that he need not suffer more than he wanted to.

The day after our talk he was discharged and I thought I would not see him again for some time. But two days later I went into the ward and ran into David.

'You're back again,' I said, surprised.

'Yes,' he said. 'I was admitted this morning. It didn't work out at home. I couldn't manage. I've realised that I can't live outside the hospital anymore. I've decided that I've had enough,' he said.

His euthanasia request had become pertinent and he had decided to ask Dr Edelman to set a date.

Later that day I asked him about the reasons for this sudden change of mind.

'Well, the thing is, I resemble something out of a . . . Steven King horror. Let me show you.' He pulled up his T-shirt. His body was bright yellow and his chest and stomach were covered with round blotches, the size of large coins. His skin was hard and scaly, reptilian.

'Err, the way I look was always very important to me.' He smiled ruefully and fell silent. 'I don't want to wait until the last moment and then have to beg for release.'

The next morning John de Wit, the ward doctor, and I went to David's room. John explained that they understood his situation, but there were rules which had to be followed. David listened in silence, nodding occasionally.

Later the same morning Dr Edelman also talked to David. I visited him in the afternoon. He was sitting next to the table, his feet up. On the table there was a packet of cigarettes.

'I just called in to see how you were doing,' I said.

'Oh, I'm alright,' he answered. 'I'm glad that everything has been arranged and I can relax now. It's a relief to know that it's all settled and that I have the certainty.' He paused. 'I still have to wait a whole week. Every night when I go to bed I hope that I won't wake up again in the morning.'

I looked it him. His face was yellow and there were blotches of Kaposi's sarcoma on his cheeks. Outside, on the street, he might have appeared monstrous, but in the context of the AIDS ward he still seemed reasonably healthy. He wasn't emaciated, he wasn't bedridden, he wasn't blind, he could still enjoy reading. I had the sudden feeling that it was too soon for him to die, that it would be a loss.

'Don't you think you're still too well to die?' I asked.

'I had a shower this morning and it almost finished me. I was exhausted. That's not how I want to go on.'

That evening I sat at home and brooded. I was haunted by the thought of David sitting there in his room, waiting. Three days later I forced myself to go to the hospital. I couldn't just let him die without having said goodbye. I drove to the hospital and climbed the stairs to the AIDS ward. It was then that I ran into Dr Edelman in the passage and he told me that it was all arranged for later that morning.

I went to David's room.

'Come on in,' he said.

'How are you feeling?' I asked.

'Alright,' he said.

'I just heard that it's all arranged for this morning,' I said.

'Yes. My mother and brother are coming at eleven. Before that Rob Edelman will come with the papers to sign and then he'll bring the cocktail at eleven thirty.'

'You can always postpone it or cancel it if you change your mind,' I said.

He paused to light a cigarette. 'No, I can't postpone it,' he said smiling, as he held out his open cigarette packet. 'I've only got enough cigarettes to last me 'till eleven thirty. If I postpone then I'll have to go down stairs again for a new packet. No, but seriously. I've seen so many people suffer. I saw the guy in the room across there suffer. I don't want to suffer like that. What for? When you know you're going to die anyway.' He fell silent, and we both stared out into the misty gloom of the winter morning.

When his mother and brother arrived I left. I returned just before Dr Edelman was due to bring the fatal cocktail. This time David was sitting up in bed. He looked well groomed. He had washed and neatly combed his hair and he wore a clean sweater. He looked tense. I walked up to the bed and stood next to him.

What do you say to someone who is about to die? 'Well,' I said nervously. 'I've come to say goodbye.'

He smiled. My throat contracted and the blood streamed to my head. I bit off my words, afraid that my voice would falter. I saw his eyes grow moist and for an instant. It lasted for a few seconds only before we regained our composure.

In the dispensary Dr Edelman was busy grinding various pills in a small mortar. He looked up as I entered.

'I'm just preparing a cocktail for David,' he said cheerfully. 'I asked him what flavour he wanted and he chose orange.' His mouth smiled, but his eyes were sad. It was a cheerfulness that I had come to recognise as masking deep despondency.

After he had dissolved the powder in some orange juice he edged past me into the passage. I followed and saw him disappear into David's room. A few minutes later he emerged and walked hurriedly down the passage before disappearing through the swinging doors into the hall. He ignored me as he passed. Later he told me that David had drunk his cocktail in a single gulp, after having smoked his last cigarette.

'You're exactly on time,' he had said when Dr Edelman arrived. 'I was down to my last cigarette.'

Now all we had to do was wait for death.

It was then that I suddenly became aware of my incongruous position. Wearing my white doctor's coat I had always been inconspicuous in the hospital. But now, standing aimlessly in the passage, I was out of place. What was I doing there anyway? What was my role? I wasn't a detached observer; not any more. But I wasn't really relevant either; I had nothing to contribute medically. I wasn't a relative. I wasn't even a friend in any real sense of the word. But I was involved, more deeply and emotionally than I had thought possible.

It took an hour before David's pulse stopped and I could go home, broken.

For me David's death was, symbolically, the last in almost two years of anthropological research on the social context in which euthanasia decisions are taken. During my research I saw more than fifty people die, their deaths often preceded by the extended agony of debilitating disease, horrible symptoms and physical decay; sometimes also by loneliness or emotional drama. David's death was not the last death that I experienced in the course of my research. But after his death I realised that I had had enough; I was tired, both physically and mentally, of the balancing act between involvement and detachment that is called anthropological fieldwork.

Being present and directly observing a social phenomenon gives us a better under-standing and more insight than simply asking about it, but having actually experi-enced it directly adds a whole new empathic dimension to that understanding. This experience can take two forms.

Firstly, it can be equivalent to what it is you are trying to understand (i.e. you actually experience what you are studying). Or, secondly, it can be partial or indirect, shedding light on the phenomenon you want to understand from a differ-ent angle. In the case above, David was dying and doctor Edelman was helping him to die; the anthropologist was doing neither, and was not about to loose a loved one. But this very equivocal experience: being close to a death and yet distant from it, poignantly enhanced his understanding of what was happening and why in a way that no questionnaire could have done.

The discussion of experience above relates to the earlier one about presence, emphasising again that fieldwork (the collection of 'data') cannot be separated from the results (the understanding that the data enables). As the anthropologist Paul Rabinow has argued, anthropology's experiential, reflective and critical activity is its strength, but it (experience) tends to be eliminated by a *positivistic* view of science that is inappropriate in a field that studies humanity (Rabinow 1977).

✐ Activity 2.3

Think about research that you have been involved in (or research that you have read about). Can you think of any direct experience of your own that has shed light on or increased you understanding of the topic in a way that would not have been possible otherwise.

Comparison and difference

Originally anthropology consisted exclusively of Western anthropologists studying non-Western, 'exotic' societies and peoples. In this context, comparison was seen as a method through which generalizations about different societies and cultures could be achieved; it was a way of making anthropology scientific. Comparison was the anthropologist's equivalent to the scientific experiment. The assumption was that the social and natural sciences could use similar approaches to study 'facts', whether natural or social.

Much has changed. Nowadays most anthropologists are no longer interested in either generalizing or being 'scientific' (whatever that might mean). Facts are no longer seen as *things* existing separately from our efforts to study them, but as constructions (see the discussion about performative ethnography above). The emphasis has shifted from generalization to description and understanding, and comparison is now concerned with difference and diversity - it is used to facilitate the understanding of culturally specific meanings rather than to achieve scientific generalization (Holy 1987).

The understanding that is sought is not only that of the *Other*, but also that of the self. Through exposure to different ways of doing things and different views on what is obvious, anthropologists have developed a critical perspective on what is considered 'normal' and 'obvious' and 'accepted' in their own culture. The anthropologist Michael Herzfeld has described anthropology as 'the study of common sense', but, as he points out, common sense 'is neither common to all cultures, nor is any version of it particularly sensible from the perspective of anyone outside its particular cultural context' (Herzfeld 2001: 1). Studying the Other gives a 'jolt' – it makes us see, suddenly, that categories, assumptions, ways of seeing that we have taken for granted, are not so obvious after all (Rhodes 1996); we find that many things we take for granted turn out not to be universals of human experience but culturally specific. This is sometimes referred to as 'studying yourself by way of the other'.

Anthropology has changed, but so has the *Other*. For one thing, anthropologists are no longer exclusively from the West, and the societies that anthropologists traditionally studied now have their own anthropologists. Anthropologists also increasingly study their own societies, doing fieldwork in hospitals, prisons, laboratories, economic institutions. Finding the *Other* nearer home is not a problem, as the '*Other*' does not refer to people from other countries or societies, but to other cultures – ways of doing and thinking that are different to what we (as researchers) take for granted. 'At its best anthropology has always been subversive. By describing different social, cultural, and psychological arrangements, it challenges commonly accepted ways of perceiving, articulating, and understanding the world' (Crapanzano 1990). This critical approach implies a degree of cultural relativism: the view that cultures should be judged on their own terms, and what is good or right or normal on one society is not necessarily so in another.

 Activity 2.4

Think about what you have just read about difference (above) and presence (as discussed earlier in this chapter). How are these related?

Anthropologists distinguish between two perspectives that are related to the issue of presence/difference: *emic* and *etic*.

- The *emic perspective* privileges the viewpoint of the local, the insider. Emic explanations are adequate if they generate statements that are real or meaningful to the people being studied.
- The *etic perspective* privileges the viewpoint of the observer, the outsider. Etic explanations tend to be formulated in terms of scientific theories.

Example: bovicide in India

In a study of the causes of death in cattle in Kerala, India, farmers insisted that because of their adherence to the Hindu prohibition against killing bovines, they would never deliberately shorten the life of their animals. However the mortality rate of male calves was more than twice that of female calves. Farmers were aware of this, and said that male calves were weaker and got sick more often. When pushed some farmers said they got sick more often because they ate less. The odd farmer suggested that they ate less because they were not permitted to drink milk from the mother for more than a few seconds. No one said that male animals were culled because there was less demand for them. (Harris 1979)

- The emics of the situation is that no one knowingly kills calves.
- The etics of the situation is that cattle sex ratios are systematically adjusted to the needs of the local economy (Harris 1979).

These concepts, which have become widely used outside anthropology, especially in social research related to health, are useful. But they are also problematic.

- There is the danger of equating emic with belief, illusion, subjective, local, traditional, and etic with knowledge, scientific fact, objective, global, modern. That is, it is difficult to avoid the impression that etic categories are somehow more real than emic ones, and that the etic perspective is somehow truer. This is clear from the example of the cows above. The message there is that they *believe* that they are not deliberately killing cattle, while we *know* that they are. In fact, emic categories are no less 'real' than etic ones.
- The distinction between emic/etic distinction can be inverted, and if we examine it critically we can argue that one person's emic is another's etic. For example, it might seem clear that the medical view that a child's convulsions are a symptom of severe malaria caused by *plasmodium falciparum* is the etic perspective, and the village mother's view that her child has been attacked by spirits is the emic view, but from the mother's point of view, theories of parasites might seem like the doctors culture-bound emic perspective, whereas explanations in terms of spirits, being part of a much wider non-biomedical aetiology, may seem obviously etic.
- It is also problematic in another sense. The local, inside perspective cannot

always be conveniently separated from the outside, expert one. Traditional and modern, Western and non-Western, local and global, cannot be separated into discrete entities. A mother might believe her child's sickness is caused by spirits, but simultaneously also believe that it is caused by parasites (see the excerpt from Haussmann Muela's study of malaria in Tanzania in Chapter 4). And the doctor may absorb local, non-biomedical ideas into his biomedical discourse. In Chapter 4 we will return to this mixing of perspectives in the discussion of syncretism.

Holism and the importance of context

Through participant observation, anthropology studies the details of what people do and why in particular settings. At the same time anthropologists assume that particular aspects of culture or particular social practices can often only be properly understood by placing them in a broader context. Anthropologists do not study isolated beliefs or behaviours in themselves, but try to understand these by placing them in the context of the local culture. However, anthropology also increasingly takes into account the fact that local societies are not isolated entities but belong to wider regional and transnational contexts, and they also increasingly include this wider context in their analyses.

For example, Paul Farmer (1997) tries to understand the dynamics of HIV and risk in Haiti by carrying out detailed ethnographic studies of vulnerable individuals and situating these in various layers of context: local culture, local and national political and economic conditions, and global relations. He criticizes the narrowly behavioural and individualistic conception of 'risk' common in epidemiology by showing how, in Haiti, a combination of gender inequality, traditional and emerging patterns of sexual union, prevalence of STDs (and lack of access to treatment for them), inadequate response by public-health authorities, lack of culturally appropriate prevention tools and political violence all contribute to particular individuals' exposure to HIV (see Chapter 7 for a detailed case study).

Thick description

Anthropologists study the complexities of social life, so the final presentation is often complex – long articles or books (ethnographies) rather than the short reports characteristic of medical journals. Clifford Geertz, following the philosopher Gilbert Ryle, has called this 'thick description'. Here is his well-cited example.

Consider two boys rapidly contracting the eyelids of their right eyes. In one, this is an involuntary twitch; in the other, a conspiratorial signal to a friend. The two movements are, as movements, identical; from an I-am-a-camera observation of them alone, one could not tell which was twitch and which was wink. Yet the difference is vast. The winker is communicating deliberately, to someone in particular, to impart a particular message, according to a socially established code, and without the knowledge of the rest of the company. The winker has done two things, contracted his eyelids and winked, while the twitcher has done only one, contracted his eyelids. Contracting your eyelids on purpose when there exists a public code in which so doing counts as a conspiratorial signal is winking.

That, however, is just the beginning. Suppose there is a third boy, who parodies the first boy's wink. He does this in the same way the second boy winked and the first twitched: by contracting his right eyelids. Only this boy is neither winking nor twitching, he is parodying someone else's attempt at winking. Here, too, a socially established code exists; and so also does a message. Only now it is not conspiracy but ridicule. If the others think he is actually winking, his whole project misfires. One can go further: uncertain of his mimicking abilities, the would-be satirist may practice at home before the mirror, in which case he is not twitching, winking, or parodying, but rehearsing; though so far as what a camera would record he is just rapidly contracting his right eyelids like all the others. The point is that between thin description of what the rehearser (parodist, winker, twitcher . . .) is doing rapidly contracting his right eyelids) and the thick description of what he is doing (practicing a burlesque of a friend faking a wink to deceive an innocent into thinking a conspiracy is in motion) lies the object of ethnography: a stratified hierarchy of meaningful structures in terms of which twitches, winks, fake-winks, parodies rehearsals of parodies are produced, perceived, and interpreted, and without which they would not in fact exist, no matter what anyone did or didn't do with his eyelids (Geertz 1973).

Thick description is not just a way of presenting 'data' in more detail. Rather, it entails the detailed investigation of webs of meaning; the presentation of the different, inter-connected contexts that are relevant for understanding the phenomenon in question. A thin description of winking an eye involves the contracting of an eyelid; a thick description distinguishes twitches from winks and identifies different kinds of winks – it includes the complex of meanings behind the actions. A thin description of lack of condom use in Rwanda might include ignorance about condoms or inadequate risk perception; a thick description would detail how condom use is embedded in a wider set of assumptions about flow and blockage, and about the body and the person (see Chapter 10).

Activity 2.5

Think about some recent social event or incident that you have experienced, or are familiar with. It may be a health-related event, for example an interaction with a doctor (or a patient if you are a health professional), or any relatively simple social situation. Try to write a short 'thick description' of this event (one or two paragraphs) exploring what you think might be the underlying meanings and wider issues that structured and influenced the event.

Summary

Anthropology involves: (a) Being present – participating, observing, interacting – in the activities being studied. As a result, anthropologists see their information as produced through interaction – praxis – rather than as neutral data that are collected like things. (b) It also entails empathic understanding through experience. (c) Through studying the *Other*, and in particular through the experience of difference, anthropology develops a critical perspective on what is considered normal, obvious and accepted. In this sense anthropology has a critical, even subversive role. (d) Phenomena cannot be understood by themselves. The wider context is important, and the many wider factors that impinge on social life need to be taken into account (symbolic systems, economic factors, politics, and so forth). (e) These various influences and strands of meaning are presented as thick description in the descriptive ethnography that is the final result of anthropological study.

References

Crapanzano V (1990) Traversing boundaries: European and North American perspectives on medical and psychiatric anthropology. *Culture, Medicine and Psychiatry* 14: 145–52.

Fabian J (1990) *Power and Performance. Ethnographic Explorations through Proverbial Wisdom and Theater in Shaba, Zaire*. Madison: University of Wisconsin Press.

Farmer P (1997) Ethnography, social analysis, and the prevention of sexually transmitted HIV infection among poor women in Haiti, in Inhorn M and Brown P (eds) *The Anthropology of Infectious Disease*. Amsterdam: Gordon & Breach.

Geertz C (1973) *The Interpretation of Cultures*. New York: Basic Books.

Harris M (1979) *Cultural Materialism: The Struggle for a Science of Culture*. New York: Random House.

Herzfeld M (2001) *Anthropology. Theoretical Practice in Culture and Society*. Oxford: Blackwell.

Holy L (1987) Introduction: description, generalization and comparison: two paradigms, in Holy L (ed) *Comparative Anthropology*. Oxford: Basil Blackwell.

Pool R (2000) *Negotiating a Good Death. Euthanasia in the Netherlands*. New York: The Haworth Press.

Rabinow P (1977) *Reflections on Fieldwork in Morocco*. Berkeley: University of California Press.

Rhodes L (1996) Studying biomedicine as a cultural system, in Sargent C and Johnson T (eds) *Medical Anthropology. Contemporary Theory and Method*. Westport: Praeger.

Tedlock D (1983) *The Spoken Word and the Work of Interpretation*. Philadelphia: University of Pennsylvania Press.

3 | Approaches to medical anthropology

Overview

In this chapter we will discuss some of the roots of medical anthropology. We will also examine some of the ways in which anthropology relates to Western scientific medicine (or biomedicine) – either collaborating to solve biomedically defined problems or critically studying biomedicine as itself a cultural phenomenon. Finally we will examine some of the important theoretical perspectives that anthropologists use to study and understand sickness, health and health care systems.

Learning objectives

By the end of this chapter you should be able to:

- **outline the main sources of medical anthropology and relate this historical background to some of the key characteristics of sociocultural anthropology**
- **identify the different ways in which anthropology interacts with medicine**
- **describe the main theoretical approaches in medical anthropology**

Key terms

Ethnomedicine This has been defined as 'those beliefs and practices relating to disease which are the products of indigenous cultural development and are not explicitly derived from the conceptual framework of modern medicine'. In the past, the term referred to the medical systems of 'primitive' or non-Western societies. However, in contemporary medical anthropology biomedicine is not uncritically privileged above other medical systems and biomedicine is also considered to be a form of ethnomedicine.

Hegemony The permeation throughout society of a system of values, attitudes, beliefs and so forth, that supports the status quo and becomes internalized to such an extent that it seems like common sense.

Definitions

According to one definition medical anthropologists

1 carry out research to comprehensively describe and interpret the biocultural interrelationships between human behaviour, past and present, and health

and disease levels, without primary regard to practical utilization of this knowledge; and

2 participate professionally in programmes whose goal is the improvement of health levels through greater understanding of the relationships between bio-sociocultural phenomena and health, and through the changing of health behaviour in directions believed to promote better health. (Foster and Anderson 1978: 10)

 Put another way, medical anthropology describes, interprets and critically appraises the relationships between culture, behaviour, health and disease, and places health and illness in the broader context of cultural, social, political, economic and historical processes.

Roots

The roots of medical anthropology are diverse, and vary depending on the approach and theoretical orientation. Some of the main sources of contemporary medical anthropology are discussed in the following section. These are early anthropological studies of ethnomedicine, the culture and personality school in anthropology, and the international public health movement (This section is based on Foster and Anderson 1978).

Studies of ethnomedicine

Even before the development of medical anthropology as a separate subdiscipline, anthropologists had collected information on illness 'beliefs and practices' in the societies they studied because they were part of culture, and also because they were seen as closely related to 'exotic' beliefs about witchcraft and sorcery.

One of these early anthropologists was WHR Rivers. In his book *Medicine, Magic and Religion* he argued that indigenous medical practices, which might seem irrational to Westerners, were rational when placed in the wider context of local beliefs and culture (Rivers 1924: 48).

This point (which seems obvious today but was not so obvious in the context of Western imperialism with its assumptions of the mental and cultural superiority of the West) was also being made by other anthropologists studying other domains. Bronislaw Malinowski, for example, in *Argonauts of the Western Pacific*, had shown that the elaborate and apparently irrational system of exchange of economically worthless goods between a group of Melanesian islands was in fact highly rational in the context of an economy of gift exchange (Malinowski 1922). And in his book *Witchcraft, Oracles and Magic Among the Azande*, EE Evans-Pritchard argued that Zande notions of witchcraft were rational if considered in the wider context of Zande aetiology (Evans-Pritchard 1937).

Although early anthropologists thought that 'primitive medicine' was rational if considered in its local cultural context, they were simultaneously convinced that it was unscientific and that its explanations were objectively incorrect. Related to this, they argued that in 'primitive' society there was a link between medicine, magic and religion (Wellin 1977; Foster and Anderson 1978: 4–8; Good 1994: 29–36).

This approach to non-Western medicine led to a number of important discussions in anthropology. It formed the basis of the 'rationality debates' from the 1960s to the 1980s (Yoder 1982). Are there universal forms of reasoning or is everything relative? Can different cultures be understood in the same way (etically), or can individual cultures only be understood from within, in their own terms (emically)? Can we distinguish between beliefs and rational scientific thought? It also led to the study of ritual and sorcery as a means of resolving social conflict, as for example in the work of Victor Turner.

Psychological anthropology and studies of culture and personality

Another group of early health-related anthropological studies focused on psychological and psychiatric phenomena. From the 1930s there was an interest in the relationship between personality and sociocultural environment.

- During this period the ideas of Freud were an important influence, and many were interested in testing whether they were universal (and therefore applicable in all cultures) or Western and culture-bound.
- The nature/nurture debate was also in full swing. Were personality traits and certain kinds of behaviour (for example, aggression) inborn and 'natural' or were they learned and therefore socially determined?
- There was interest in the so-called 'culture bound syndromes'. These were disorders – mainly mental disorders – that were thought to exist only in specific cultures, or at least take on culturally specific forms. For example *amok*, which involves violent and murderous attacks, using a traditional *kris* (dagger), by middle-aged Malay men following a period of brooding over some insult.
- The universality of Western psychiatric categories (for example, schizophrenia) was being questioned: were disorders such as schizophrenia universal or were they Western and culture bound?

International public health

Although the Rockerfeller Foundation has been involved in international public health since early in the twentieth century, it was only during the Second World War that the US government initiated collaborative health projects in Latin America. In the postwar period these were extended to Asia and Africa. With the founding of the World Health Organization (WHO) major bilateral and multilateral health programmes became common. In these international and cross-cultural contexts it soon became clear to health workers that many health problems were as much social and cultural phenomena as they were biological.

Here anthropologists were seen as the obvious people to inform health professionals about how traditional beliefs and practices conflicted with biomedical assumptions, how social and cultural factors influence health and health-seeking behaviour.

In the 1950s many international public health projects welcomed anthropologists. Anthropology was seen as providing insight into why some programmes were less successful than had been hoped, and it was not threatening to health professionals because it defined problems of resistance as lying with recipient peoples. Foster and Anderson see the international public health movement as the major root of medical anthropology (Foster and Anderson 1978).

Activity 3.1

Reread the section on comparison and difference in Chapter 2. How does that relate to what you have just read about the work of the early studies of ethnomedicine?

Feedback

The early studies of ethnomedicine were very much in the older comparative tradition. Other medical systems were considered interesting because they were different and exotic, and their practices were rational within the context of local culture, but the assumption was always that they were inferior to Western biomedicine in more universal and objective terms. The experience of difference did not have the effect on these early anthropologists of getting them to reflect critically on the assumptions and values of their own medical system.

Theoretical and applied medical anthropology

Part of the anthropological interest in health and illness is theoretically motivated: understanding health and illness as a major category of culture (for example, the early ethnomedical studies). But much of the anthropology in the context of international public health from the 1950s has been carried out in collaboration with health workers and aimed at improving health. Indeed, the first major survey of the field was titled 'Applied anthropology in medicine' (Caudill 1953).

- *Applied medical anthropology* is aimed at solving health problems in particular settings. This is usually carried out in collaboration with biomedical health professionals.
- *Theoretical medical anthropology* is aimed at understanding the functioning of medical systems as cultural phenomena, and developing more general theories about underlying processes.

A similar distinction is made between anthropology *of* medicine and anthropology *in* medicine.

- Anthropology *in* medicine: anthropologists work together with health professionals to solve problems that are defined by the latter (for example, why don't people at risk of HIV use condoms?).
- Anthropology *of* medicine: anthropologists take medicine (including biomedicine) as an object of study and define the relevant topics and approach (for example, what non-medical factors influence how doctors make end-of-life decisions?). This is explored further in Chapter 8, and in the final chapters of the book.

Some think that they are incompatible: anthropology of medicine would loose its critical edge if it identified too closely with biomedicine and its priorities; and if it became too critical of biomedicine, anthropology in medicine would become bogged down by relativism and theory, which would alienate medical anthropologists from medical colleagues and render them incapable of contributing to the solution of health problems. Others think the distinction is largely analytic, with applied work feeding data back into theory and theory having value in practical settings.

In practice, applied medical anthropology tends to be mainly anthropology *in* biomedicine because of the dominant position of biomedicine and the unequal power relations between doctors and anthropologists in health care and medical research settings. In such settings doctors define the problems and the research priorities and anthropologists tend to play an ancillary role. Related to this, those in charge of medical research are often reluctant to allow anthropologists to focus on medical research and the medical research setting itself as part of the object of study (for example the interaction between medical research and local communities) because they find this either threatening or irrelevant (we will come back to this in Chapters 11 and 12). One way of viewing this is to see anthropology *of* medicine as part of *anthropology*, and anthropology *in* medicine as part of *medicine* (see Chapter 7 for further discussion).

Theoretical approaches in medical anthropology

Medical anthropologists make use of different theoretical approaches when studying and interpreting health and sickness. In the extract below, taken from a paper by Paul Farmer and Byron Good, the four main theoretical approaches in medical anthropology are discussed (Farmer and Good 1991). The article from which this abridged extract was taken appeared in a book written mainly for psychologists entitled *Mental Representation in Health and Illness*, which goes some way to explaining their emphasis on illness representation.

 Activity 3.2

While reading the extract, pay particular attention to what the authors say about the 'enlightenment model'.

Four anthropological approaches to the study of illness representations

Illness representations as folk beliefs: the applied tradition
Since the 1950s, anthropologists have collaborated with public health professionals in a wide variety of projects designed to bring services to populations in developing societies and in the United States. Much of this work focused on a deceptively complex problem: how to get local populations to alter their behaviour in a fashion that would improve their health. Wells can be dug, vaccinations offered, but if these services and technologies are not used or not used appropriately, they will be of little value. Public health officials saw resistance to such obviously effective behaviours as irrational, the result of ignorance, superstitions, or traditional views that conflict with

modern medical knowledge and require change. Social psychologists of the same era, collaborating with health specialists facing similar problems, were developing the Health Belief Model as a research and intervention tool. Anthropologists, such as Benjamin Paul addressed the problem by analysing health beliefs in relation to a local culture.

Indigenous 'items of belief,' Paul argued, must be understood from the 'native's point of view.' Only then can the seemingly irrational be understood, and only then can programs of education be developed that work within the local frame of reference.

Many of the anthropological contributions to public health work begin with this important, if rather straightforward, set of insights, However, this general approach to the study of illness representations has limitations from both practical and theoretical points of view. First, the behaviours identified are often best understood in relation to structural conditions – gross inequalities, poverty, inferior housing and work conditions – or the irrationalities of health bureaucracies and practitioners, rather than as a result of rational albeit mistaken beliefs. Very often neither the 'beliefs' nor the behaviours are under the voluntary control of individuals, as this 'Enlightenment' model assumes.

Second, facile recourse to the label 'belief' has been challenged on methodological grounds. Items termed beliefs are often deduced from illness narratives, which have been found to vary by social context, the audience of the narrative, and the stage in the illness process in which the account is elicited. Illness stories told to a doctor differ from those told to friends in the home, and both differ from those told to a researcher. It is far from clear that this story represents 'belief.'

Third, the very concept 'belief' as a frame for analysing illness representations has been challenged on theoretical grounds. 'Beliefs' in 20th-century philosophy, have been conceived as propositional, normative, and voluntary. Beliefs are often represented as a set of propositions which can be judged as more or less true, depending on the adequacy of their ostensive representation of the objective world. Folk beliefs about illness are, from this perspective, a kind of protoscience, with medical science providing the norm against which they may be judged. Indeed, since the 18th century 'belief' has increasingly been used in Western languages for propositions that either are essentially uncertain or are not true.

The view that the earth is round is knowledge, not belief. Inquiry into folk 'beliefs' thus assumes biomedicine as the norm, authorizing the perspective of the researcher over that of the research subject. Furthermore, this generally rationalist perspective assumes that *beliefs drive behaviour*, that individuals weigh the costs and benefits of particular acts based on their beliefs about the threats and potential consequences of behaviour, and that they seek to maximize benefits in their behaviour. Behaviour, as well as beliefs, are thus essentially voluntary characteristics of individuals seeking to maximize their personal good.

The theory of illness representations as folk beliefs has been criticized on several grounds.

It is far from clear that beliefs are propositional in form or indeed that believing, as we conceive this process, is a universal phenomenon. Opinions and the speech acts from which they are deduced are seldom protoscientific, and the 'objective reality' to which they refer is not simply the biological world but a socially and culturally constituted reality. A concept of belief that authorizes the knowledge of the researcher over the opinions of those who are the object of study is thus open to epistemological criticism. It also poses subtle methodological problems that challenge the validity of the findings. As Favret-Saada remarks, when a Parisian intellectual asks a French peasant 'Do you believe in witchcraft?' the only response possible is 'Of course not, do you take me for a fool?' (Favret-Saada 1980). Finally, the 'rational man' theory of motivation and behaviour is inadequate, even when rationality is treated as a culturally distinctive form of reasoning.

Psychologists as well as anthropologists are increasingly aware of the psychological and structural conditions that undermine the relation between rational understanding and human behaviour. Although serious questions have been raised about the view of illness representations as folk beliefs, this tradition of applied research has continued vitality, contributes in an extremely important way to efforts to solve global health problems, and is likely to play an ongoing role in applied research. However, the recognition of the theoretical and methodological problems outlined here have contributed to the development of alternative approaches in the field.

Illness representations as formal cognitive structures: the view from cognitive anthropology

Researchers working within the cognitive paradigm have focused on the formal structures of cognitive processing. Within the anthropological tradition, these are viewed as representational forms provided by culture, and an elegant tradition of formal methods has developed to investigate how these forms vary from society to society as well as among individuals.

Some early research in this paradigm focused on medical classification: symptoms of illness, diseases, causes of illness, and types of healers. Culture, it was argued, identifies the distinctive features of such phenomena and provides frames for organizing relations among them. Detailed studies were undertaken to investigate the relations between representations of illness and patterns of health-care seeking. This tradition has been productive and continues to generate research investigating cultural models of particular disorders, their cross-cultural variation, and levels of consensus about them among individuals within a culture.

Some cognitivists have begun to focus on illness narratives, their cultural shaping, and the cultural models that underlie their production. Such work has begun to shift attention from the formal properties of illness models to their relation to natural discourse, and thus to context and performance characteristics of illness representations. This growing interest they share with sociolinguists, interpretive anthropologists, and others interested in illness narratives.

Cognitive anthropologists have provided elegant methods and analyses of folk illness beliefs. Their work has shared some of the criticisms, however, of the less methodologically developed approach to illness beliefs in the applied tradition, outlined previously. In particular, illness representations have continued to be seen in mentalistic terms, abstracted from 'embodied knowledge,' affect, and social and historical forces that shape illness meanings. Illness models are viewed in formal, semantic terms, with little attention to pragmatic and performative dimensions. And the formal methods that lie at the heart of their contribution often raise the specter of artifact, the danger that the methods *produce* the neat cognitive models claimed to be those of the informants or produce a form of illness representations that is highly constrained by the mode of their elicitation.

Illness representations as culturally constituted illness realities: the 'meaning-centered' tradition

Arthur Kleinman's work, beginning in the late 1970s, marked the emergence of medical anthropology as a systematic and theoretically grounded field of inquiry within the larger discipline. Kleinman designated the medical system a 'cultural system,' and thus a distinctive field of anthropological inquiry. His work combined an interest in complex medical systems, detailed ethnographic analyses of illness and healing in Chinese cultures, theoretical development linked to symbolic, interpretive, and social constructivist writing, and an interest in applied medical anthropology. Here we briefly outline some dimensions of the work on illness representations that have grown out of this tradition.

Kleinman argued that illness representations can be understood as 'explanatory models,' schemata for understanding illness held by individual sufferers and families as well as clinicians and healers, models available in popular, folk, and professional medical cultures. These models shed light on questions concerning etiology, type and onset of symptoms, pathophysiology, course and consequences of illness, and appropriate treatments. In contrast with cognitive researchers, who tended to rely on formal elicitation techniques, researchers investigating explanatory models often conducted their studies in 'clinically relevant' contexts, among the sick and those they consulted during illness or therapeutic interventions. Explanatory models were recognized to emerge in situated discourse, to shift with course of illness, to constitute personal accounts of various dimensions of the illness experience.

Thus research in this tradition tended to be concerned less with the way in which people store and process information about sickness and more with ways in which explanatory models come into play as people attempt to interpret disturbing somatic, psychological, or social experience. Explanatory model research has probed the place of such models in discourse about illness and their role in the elaboration of 'illness realities' and the shaping of responses to such realities in the context of socially organized power relations.

Second, practitioners of the meaning-centered approach resisted the formal definition of illness categories in relation to distinctive features, exploring instead the notion that illness representations are multi vocal symbols that condense a set of associated meanings and are linked to an underlying 'semantic network.'

The anthropological account of semantic networks treats them as *cultural*, as symbols associated at a deep level in culture, associations which both underlie explanatory models and social experience and are built up through historical practice and experience. Although no single formal method has been developed to study semantic networks, studies have been conducted of 'heart distress' in Iran, and 'bad blood' in Haiti.

Third, drawing on phenomenological and social constructionist theories, medical anthropologists have explored the relation between illness representations and illness 'realities.' That which is real for members of a society – 'diseases' treated by physicians, possessing spirits, – are constituted through representational and interpretive processes.

The nature of those realities, though often highly contested, is determined not only by the natural history of biological and psychological processes, both of which may play a more or less important role, but also by the representation of illness. Research has thus focused on the role of rhetorical processes in the construction and reconstruction of illness realities, on the relation of representation to embodied experience, on the historical production, continuity, and change of illness representations, and on the representation of illness realities in narratives.

The approach to illness representations outlined here has led to debate both among its practitioners and among those outlining alternative approaches. Explanatory model research has been criticized along lines outlined for the folk belief model as assuming a 'rational man,' although from the beginning explanatory models were seldom seen as fixed models motivating behaviour. On the other hand, the methods of the approach are essentially ethnographic and lack the experimental rigor of the cognitivists; they have also been criticized from that perspective. More recently, some have charged that the view that illness realities are constituted through interpretive and representational processes treats such realities as consensual and fails to provide a 'critical' stance vis-à-vis illness representations. Some have begun to develop this position as an alternative theoretical frame for the analysis of illness representations.

Illness representations as authorized misrepresentation: views from 'critical' medical anthropology

In contrast to the social constructionist line, some have attempted to develop a neo-Marxist approach to illness representations. One touchstone to the position is Antonio Gramsci's analysis of hegemony and the development of his claim that common sense is ultimately hegemonic, a view of reality developed to justify existing social relations.

A critical medical anthropology forcefully poses the question of when illness representations are actually *misrepresentations* that serve the interests of those in power, be they colonial powers, elites within a society, the medical profession, or empowered men. Forms of suffering grounded in social relations can be defined as illness, medicalised, and brought under the authority of the medical profession and the state. Thus symptoms of hunger or diseases that result from poverty, whether among the North American poor or the impoverished cane cutters of Brazil, are medicalised, treated as a condition of individual bodies – 'diarrhoea,' 'TB,' 'nerves,' or 'stress' rather than a collective concern. The transformation of a political problem into a medical one is often akin to 'neutralizing' critical consciousness and thus serves the interests of the hegemonic class. Analysis of illness representations therefore requires a critical unmasking of the dominant interests, an expose of the mechanisms by which they are supported by authorized discourse: What is misrepresented in illness representations must be revealed.

Idioms of distress and illness representations of those who are suffering may, in turn, be viewed as forms of resistance. Here the critical task would seem to be offering an interpretation of an illness that renders explicit the social and political meanings locked inside a sickness.

In short, critical analysis must examine how illness representations serve to represent and misrepresent power relations within a society. Development of this approach follows in part a shift within anthropology from a dominant focus on symbols and meaning to a focus on practice. These ideas have not yet been fully explored within medical anthropology. However, they are certain to continue to serve as the nexus for debate about the nature of illness representations.

Now answer the following questions:

1 What do the authors mean by the 'enlightenment model'?
2 How do the authors criticize this model?
3 What are the methodological and practical consequences of this when doing medical or epidemiological research?

Feedback

1 Basically, that people's beliefs determine their behaviour in a direct and rational fashion, and that we can understand behaviour (and change it) if we know and understand the underlying beliefs.

2 First, beliefs do not drive behaviour in any simple one-to-one way. Behaviour is often determined by structural constraints such as poverty, discrimination and bureaucracy, rather than simply being the result of beliefs (we will return to this in Chapters 6 and 7). Second, what are described as people's 'beliefs' have often been abstracted from the contexts of the narrative discourse of which they were part and the specific setting in which that discourse was generated. For example, stories of illness told to a doctor differ from those told to friends, and both differ from those told to a researcher; and stories vary before and after diagnosis. Third, the word 'belief' implies a statement that is not true (as when belief is opposed to knowledge). As a result, studying local 'beliefs' already implies that the biomedical perspective of the researcher is the correct one.

3 Standardized instruments such as survey questionnaires produce a standard set of decontextualized local beliefs. This raises questions about the validity of sociocultural data (remember the reporting of the frequency of euthanasia requests in the example in Chapter 1). It also points to the problems inherent in the practice of designing health interventions based on surveys of 'attitudes and beliefs'.

Summary

Medical anthropology has diverse roots, depending on the approach and theoretical orientation. Some of the main sources of contemporary medical anthropology are: the early anthropological studies of ethnomedicine, the culture and personality school in anthropology, and the international public health movement.

In order to understand the relationship between anthropology and medicine, a distinction is often made between anthropology *in* medicine and anthropology *of* medicine. In the former anthropologists work together with biomedical health professionals to solve problems that are defined by the latter; in the latter anthropologists take medicine (including biomedicine) as an object of study.

Medical anthropology makes use of a number of theoretical perspectives, some mainly on the side of anthropology in medicine and others more in vogue in the anthropology of medicine. The applied tradition focuses mainly on studying illness beliefs with the aim of contributing to health interventions. The cognitive approach is interested in revealing and describing the underlying cultural codes and schemas that structure people's interpretations of illness. The meaning-centred tradition focuses on the emic perspective of patients in an attempt to understand their experience of suffering. Finally, the critical perspective places emphasis on the wider structural factors that determine health and illness and the powerful interests that maintain these.

References

Caudill W (1953) Applied anthropology in medicine, in Kroeber AL (ed) *Anthropology Today: An Encyclopedic Inventory*. Chicago: University of Chicago Press.

Evans-Pritchard EE (1937) *Witchcraft, Oracles and Magic Among the Azande*. Oxford: Oxford University Press.

Farmer P and Good BJ (1991) Illness representations in medical anthropology: a critical review and case study of the representation of AIDS in Haiti, in Skelton J and Croyle R (eds) *Mental Representation in Health and Illness*. New York: Springer Verlag.

Favret-Saada J (1980) *Deadly Words. Witchcraft in the Bocage*. Cambridge: Cambridge University Press.

Foster GM and Anderson BG (1978) *Medical Anthropology*. New York: Wiley.

Good BJ (1994) *Medicine, Rationality and Experience. An Anthropological Perspective*. Cambridge: Cambridge University Press.

Kleinman A, Eisenberg L and Good B (1978) Culture, illness and care. Clinical lessons from anthropologic and cross-cultural research. *Annals of Internal Medicine* 88: 251–8.

Malinowski B (1922) *Argonauts of the Western Pacific*. London: Routledge & Kegan Paul.

Rivers WHR (1924) *Medicine, Magic and Religion*. London: Routledge.

Wellin E (1977) Theoretical orientations in medical anthropology: continuity and change over half a century, in Landy D (ed) *Culture, Disease and Healing. Studies in Medical Anthropology*. London: Macmillan.

Yoder PS (1982) Issues in the study of ethnomedical systems in Africa, in *African Health and Healing Systems*. Los Angeles: Crossroads Press.

4 Medical systems and medical syncretism

Overview

In this chapter we discuss medical systems, often considered to be the main object of medical anthropology. We will examine Arthur Kleinman's influential model of medical systems and then go on to present some of the main criticisms of this approach. We then discuss the notion of medical pluralism and the criticism of this, and present an alternative approach that is based more in practice and practical situations and regards medical systems as syncretic rather than plural. The chapter ends with an extended case study of medical syncretism in relation to malaria in Tanzania.

Learning objectives

By the end of this chapter you should be able to:

- describe the main characteristics of medical systems and critically evaluate the concept of medical system
- understand the concept of syncretism
- explain how popularization and indigenization contribute to the syncretization of medical traditions
- discuss and critically evaluate the concept of medicalization

Key terms

Functionalism The theory that society is a unitary whole and that the parts all contribute to the maintenance of the whole. The existence of behaviours or social institutions, and the form they take, are explained in terms of their contribution to the stability of society as a whole.

Indigenization This term usually applies to the process of adaptation to the local social and cultural environment that Western biomedicine undergoes when it becomes part of non-Western medical systems. However, it could also refer to the inclusion of aspects of non-Western medical traditions into biomedicine (for example, acupuncture).

Medicalization The extension of biomedicine into areas of life that previously were considered social rather than medical (for example, birth and dying), and the expansion of the power and influence of medical experts, sometimes even to the extent that medicine takes on a deviance control function (for instance, in child-abuse cases).

Medical pluralism The existence, within one medical system, or one society, of different medical traditions.

Popularization When aspects of a professional medical tradition (usually biomedicine) filter down into the popular sector (for example, the informal sale of antibiotics, back street injectionists). It could also refer to the popular use of aspects of other medical traditions (for example the sale of Ayurvedic teas and remedies in British supermarkets).

Syncretism A term taken from religious studies, refers to unifying or reconciling different or opposing schools of thought.

Medical systems

The object of medical anthropology is often considered to be ethnomedical systems. A medical system is a community's ideas and practices relating to illness and health. Medical systems are not entities but conceptual models developed by researchers to enable them to understand how people deal with health and illness in particular cultural settings. (Remember the discussion of reification in relation to the concept of culture in Chapter 1.)

The medical doctor and anthropologist Arthur Kleinman developed what is probably the most comprehensive theory of medical systems (he calls them health care systems) in his book *Patients and Healers in the Context of Culture* (Kleinman 1980). He writes that 'The health care system includes people's beliefs (largely tacit and unaware of the system as a whole) and patterns of behaviour. Those beliefs and behaviours are governed by cultural rules' (Kleinman 1980: 26). (Note the holistic approach and the idea of culture as underlying code.)

Kleinman identifies three sectors of medical systems.

The professional sector

This consists of the 'organized healing professions', which, according to Kleinman, usually take a modern biomedical approach, although in some societies they also include indigenous professional medical traditions, such as Ayurveda in India and classical Chinese medicine (Leslie 1976; Kleinman 1980: 53–9). Where Western scientific medicine becomes part of non-Western medical systems it often undergoes a process of *indigenization*, adapting to its local social and cultural environment. A related process is *popularization*, in which aspects of scientific medicine filter down into the popular sector.

Biomedicine has become dominant to such an extent that it is often considered to be the only relevant aspect of medical systems, and public health problems and priorities (and the focus of research) are determined exclusively by biomedicine. (See the discussion of anthropology of/in medicine and the subordinate role of anthropology in health research settings in Chapter 3.) As a result 'the solutions offered fit professionally sanctioned solution-frames and are evaluated only from that standpoint' (Kleinman 1980: 56). Because they are socialized into a biomedical subculture that they have internalized and which they can no longer view critically (remember the discussion of culture in Chapter 1, and the concept of hegemony in Chapter 3), biomedical insiders often take their own view as objective and reject local and lay interpretations of sickness and health as unscientific. Kleinman lists a number of dogmas that are related to this view (Kleinman 1980: 57):

- Health-related activities undertaken by patients themselves or other sectors of the medical system are dangerous.
- The biological aspects of health problems are 'real' and the psychosocial and cultural aspects are second order.
- The relationship between doctor and patient (and relatives) is one between experts and those who are ignorant; the doctor's role is to give instructions and the patient is expected to comply. (We will discuss the issue of adherence in more detail.)

The extension of biomedicine into wider areas of life and the expansion of the power and influence of medical experts is known as *medicalization*. Childbirth is an example of this: what used to be a natural process that occurred at home is now a medicalized process that in many countries is sanctioned only in a medical institution under the supervision of medical experts. Western countries, such as the Netherlands, where home birth is encouraged, are the exception.

The folk or traditional sector

The folk sector, according to Kleinman, is the non-professional, non-bureaucratic, specialist sector of health care that overlaps with the professional sector at the one extreme and the lay sector at the other. Sometimes a distinction is made between 'sacred' and 'secular' aspects of folk healing. The former involves the use of supernatural forces (shamanism, ritual), the latter is non-supernatural (herbalism, bone-setting).

Needless to say, the different categories are porous and it is sometimes difficult to fit particular kinds of healers clearly into one sector. In *Patients and Healers*, Kleinman's ethnographic material comes from his extensive work in Taiwan. He describes the professional sector, which consists of Western-style biomedical doctors and Chinese-style doctors, and the folk sector, consisting of shamans (*tâng-kis*). In between these are the herbalists and bonesetters. These two latter categories illustrate that, in this setting, the essential difference between folk and professional sectors relates to government recognition and professional organization.

The popular sector

The popular sector is the largest part of the medical system and the least studied, according to Kleinman. People's medical choices are rooted in popular culture and when they have received treatment from the folk or professional sector they go back to the popular sector to evaluate and decide what to do next. The popular sector interacts with the other sectors while they are often isolated from each other.

According to Kleinman, the conventional view is that professionals organize health care for lay people. In fact, he argues, what happens is that lay people activate their health care by deciding when and whom to consult, whether to adhere, whether treatment is effective, when to switch to another treatment, and so forth (Kleinman 1980: 51).

Similarly, in relation to the discussion about adherence (also known as compliance or convergence), James Trostle points out that labelling patients non-adherent because they follow their own ideas about treatment misses the point: this is what people have always done. The idea of 'non-adherence' equates a temporary constellation of power relationships (between doctors and patients) with the medical system more generally, ignoring more universal forms of obtaining care: self-management. That is, the popular sector is primary and what is normal behaviour in that sector becomes labelled as non-adherent once the patient's actions are reinterpreted in the context of the professional sector (Trostle 1988).

Activity 4.1

Read this extract from Kleinman's *Patients and Healers* (Kleinman 1980: 159–60).

Since psychological disorders among Chinese fit better into the somatic treatment orientation of Western-style and Chinese-style medical practice than into the psychotherapeutic orientation of psychiatry, it is not surprising that we find psychiatric practice with Chinese patients frequently following a medical rather than a psychotherapeutic treatment approach. Nonetheless, psychotherapy increasingly appeals to the younger and better educated in Taiwan, who have assimilated Western values and are quite 'modern' in most regards, notwithstanding that psychotherapeutic treatment services are still not widely available there. Yet even among this elite group, psychotherapy must be practiced in a special manner that makes sense within the Chinese cultural context. It needs to be more directed and supportive and less insight-oriented. It cannot be separated from general medical questions and procedures. And it must be extremely sensitive to culturally shaped coping mechanisms for managing dysphoric affect and behavioural norms. Of all the coping mechanisms, somatisation is perhaps the most difficult problem to manage in psychotherapy with Chinese patients. Most patients with somatisation often remain unconvinced that their problems are psychological rather than medical (and indeed their illness is 'medical'). They see little reason to talk about issues that are personal. Many are simply unable to define or articulate personal problems in psychological terms, and they do not believe that talk therapy without medication can be effective or worth paying for. Because these illness beliefs and behaviours are sanctioned by Chinese culture, they are especially hard to deal with effectively in psychotherapy. Morita therapy was developed by a Japanese psychiatrist to provide a culturally appropriate psychological treatment, oriented away from intrapsychic analysis and self-preoccupation and toward the control of external behaviour, for a neurotic disorder among Japanese, *shinkeishitsu* (neurasthenia), which involves somatisation. Unfortunately, in Chinese culture there is no analogy to date of this 'indigenisation' of psychotherapy, which constructs a modern cultural fit between illness and its treatment – unless work 'therapy' and self-criticism in the People's Republic of China can be viewed in this way.

What is the indigenization that Kleinman is describing here? Write down some examples of indigenization from your own experience.

Feedback

The indigenization here is the way in which Western psychotherapy is somatized and made more 'medical' in China. This is because the symptoms that a Western physician would consider to be the somatization of an underlying psychological disorder are seen by patients as physically based (even younger and more educated patients among whom psychotherapy is popular).

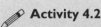 **Activity 4.2**

1 Write down some examples, from your experience, of the popularization of biomedicine.
2 Medicalization is the spread of biomedicine into ever wider areas of social life (for example, childbirth). Think of some other examples of medicalization. Why have they developed? What problems do they bring with them? How could they be reduced?

 Feedback

1 For example:

- Popular notions of cholesterol and heart disease, the use of equipment to check blood pressure, popular ideas about germs and various measures to counter them.
- The widespread use of injections by non-biomedical practitioners, often in a way that would be unacceptable to a biomedical physician.

2 For example, the medicalization of child abuse through the increasing involvement of medical 'experts'. Problem: the power of medical experts extends beyond medicine and into the social realm. Solution: keep power and influence of medical experts limited and open to critical scrutiny, involve other disciplines – for example, the involvement of anthropology in a child abuse scandal in the UK in the 1990s resulted in the debunking of accusations of abuse in the context of satanic rituals (Fontaine 1998).

Criticism of the concept of medical systems

The concept of medical systems is widely used in medical anthropology and it is useful in helping us to understand various aspects of how society deals with health and illness, but it is also problematic.

- In discussions of medical systems, especially in the older literature, there was an underlying assumption that components of the system exist, or have taken on their current form, because they fulfil some function within the whole. In other words, the fact that they exist implies that they are useful, that they must contribute to the maintenance of the society of which they are part. This is referred to as *functionalism*. For example, in the quotation from Foster and Anderson above, medical systems are described as consisting of knowledge, beliefs and practices relating to health that 'promote optimum functioning of society'.

- The term 'system' suggests unity and integration whereas, in practice, the ways in which people deal with health and illness, and the ways in which medical 'systems' work, are often far from integrated and systematic, and often messy, chaotic and indeterminate. In this regard, the anthropologist Murray Last has referred to 'non-systems' (Last 1981). Indeed, Kleinman, in his later work, has himself been critical of the concept of the medical system, with its suggestion of formal structures and innate divisions, and he has distanced himself from the functionalist aspects of his earlier work (Kleinman 1995).

From pluralism to syncretism

The idea of medical systems is closely related to the concept of *medical pluralism*, the use, within one system, or one society, of different sectors or medical traditions. This can take different forms:

- Separate use. For example, African villagers generally go to a health centre for the treatment of gonorrhoea and to a diviner if they suspect witchcraft.
- Hierarchy of resort. In Africa this often takes the form of initial self-medication followed by biomedical treatment if the former does not work and finally traditional treatment if the sickness does not respond to biomedicine. In Europe this may take the form of initial consultation of a biomedical doctor followed by the use of alternative forms of treatment or self-medication if the disease turns out to be chronic or declared incurable by the doctor.
- Simultaneous use. People use different kinds of treatment at the same time. For example, John Janzen describes people who think that biomedicine is effective, 'but their conviction that less tangible social and mystical causes have intervened obliges them to intersperse visits to the hospital with visits to indigenous practitioners' (Janzen 1978).

In fact, as the last point suggests, what we have in practice is not so much medical pluralism but *syncretism*. Syncretism, a term taken from religious studies, refers to unifying or reconciling different or opposing schools of thought.

The sectors of the medical system are not always as clearly distinguished as the discussion of medial systems above suggests, and reality is usually much more messy. For one thing, there is no such thing as 'pure' traditional medicine, local aetiologies and so forth (see the discussion of popularization and indigenization above). 'Tradition' is itself a problematic concept, and what we refer to as tradition is continually being reconstructed and reinterpreted (Hobsbawm and Ranger 1983). This applies equally to biomedicine, which is itself a form of ethnomedicine, steeped in culture and continually changing. For example, Cecil Helman has shown how ideas from pre-biomedical medicine are not only central in how patients in England interpret illnesses like the common cold, but also infiltrate doctors' explanations (Helman 1978). And anyone who has had experience of medical treatment in different countries will have noticed that there are differences in the way biomedicine is practised in, say, Europe and Africa or, within Europe, between the Netherlands and France (for example, in the willingness or reluctance to prescribe antibiotics and the speed with which doctors resort to third-line antibiotics). As Murray Last has pointed out, rather than a pluralistic system, there is (at least from the patient's point of view) often a 'single, wide-ranging corpus of illnesses for which all the different healers between them should possess a cure' (Last 1981).

What this suggests is that rather than trying to reveal 'systems' we should focus on studying practice (what people actually do when they are ill or suffer misfortune). Health-seeking behaviour is not simply the enactment of 'beliefs' within the confines of a 'culture' or a 'system', but a creative process in which we must recognize the role of invention, innovation, and disorder. Johannes Fabian has characterized this approach as 'theorising from below' (Fabian 1985) (see also the discussion of performative ethnography in Section 1, Chapter 1).

Activity 4.3

Read the abridged extract from *Fake malaria and hidden parasites – the ambiguity of malaria*, by Susanna Haussman Muela et al. (2000), focusing on the ambiguity of malaria and how syncretism relating to malaria is expressed in this community. It has been taken from a report of an 18-month anthropological study of malaria treatment seeking behaviour in south eastern Tanzania. Malaria is highly endemic and perennial, and the most commonly diagnosed disease and the leading cause of mortality for children under five in this area.

Local knowledge about malaria

The local model of malaria mainly consists of elements derived from the biomedical model, although the two are not entirely congruent. We have written 'malaria' in italics when we specifically refer to the local model.

The inhabitants have been exposed to health education for more than 20 years and have a good biomedical knowledge of malaria transmission. In the questionnaire, 98% mentioned mosquito bites as the cause of *malaria*. Some, however, also referred to other modes of transmission, namely drinking or wading through dirty water or being exposed to 'intensive sun'.

Malaria is felt to be a common, everyday illness that means a big health burden to the whole population. The most frequently reported symptom for *malaria* is *homa*, which literally translated means fever. However, the notion of *homa* has a broader meaning and is also commonly used for expressing general malaise or diffuse body pains.

While *homa* is mandatory, a broad range of other signs and symptoms are enumerated as manifestations of *malaria*: severe headache, joint pains, chills, yellowish vomiting, diarrhoea, stomach ache, convulsions, general body weakness, loss of appetite, 'the child does not play' and dizziness. Although malaria often presents in a mild form, people are well aware of its possible severe consequences, especially in children. In the questionnaire, practically all mothers (99%) affirmed that if untreated, the child can die of *malaria*, and 87% stated that death can occur within hours or a few days.

Complications of malaria are recognized, but included in the interpretative model of two common 'folk illnesses' of children, *degedege* (convulsions) and *bandama* (splenomegaly and severe anaemia).

Treatment of *malaria* with pharmaceuticals is preferred to home treatment with local herbs or traditional therapies. Administration of western drugs in the home is widely practiced: 81% of the respondents said that they would first treat their child with antipyretics or antimalarials before attending the hospital. People habitually speak of *malaria* as a 'normal illness' (*ugonjwa wa kawaida*) or an 'illness of God' (*ugonjwa wa Mungu*) meaning that it belongs to the natural order created by God. 'Normal illnesses' exclude any ailments resulting from intentional actions of witches (*wachawi*) or spirits (*mashetani*).

The witches' crafts
Belief in witchcraft (*uchawi*) is widespread in Tanzania. In the study area most informants affirmed that they have been in contact with it. The traditional healers have the skills to detect and treat witchcraft, and the power to protect their clients from witchcraft. While for 'normal illnesses' people generally state that the 'Europeans' have better medicine, in cases of witchcraft, western medicine is not only inadequate, but can even aggravate the condition.

Rethinking illness: the ambiguity of malaria
People have a clear concept of cause, symptomatology and treatment of *malaria*. However, in actual illness episodes, they are confronted with the ambiguity of malaria. Firstly, because the symptomatology of malaria itself is ambiguous. The manifestations of malaria are variable and its symptoms often diffuse, making a differential diagnosis based on the clinical presentation difficult. Secondly, because absolutely identical symptomatologies can be equally well explained using different interpretative models that coexist in the local cultural repertoire, i.e. 'malaria' and 'witchcraft'. This makes a causal attribution based on the observation of symptoms impossible. The question then is which interpretation is 'selected' among different possibilities? With the onset of *homa* ('fever'), the most usual interpretation is initially to think of a 'normal' illness (usually *malaria*). People explicitly recognize this association, but as a first orientation only. They can by no means be certain of it before the disease is diagnosed and successfully treated by a specialist.

Other possible interpretations set in when the model of *malaria* does not provide satisfactory explanations for all events that occur during illness. In filling in the gaps, people call upon available knowledge which transcends the limitations of the model.

Characteristic indicators for witchcraft are when the disease cannot be detected at the hospital, or when antimalarial treatment does not provide the expected relief. Suspicions are reinforced when unusual signs coincide with the development of the disease. This is illustrated by the account of a mother who one morning found her son with high fever and noticed peculiar scratches on his skin. These she interpreted as the marks of the witch's claws left behind after the attack.

Since illness experiences are inextricably embedded within people's lifeworld, rethinking illness takes place within a broader situational framework. Speculations about malevolent intrusions mainly arise in the context of social conflicts, when a series of misfortunes in the family occurs or when somebody already has a long history of witchcraft experiences. The following case gives an example of how existing social tensions result in witchcraft accusation after illness has not responded to hospital treatment.

The informant had lived together with her husband for several years. When she was pregnant with her sixth child, her husband left her and went to live with another partner. After the child's birth, however, he decided to return to his wife and to take care of his family. This, in turn, upset the mother of the abandoned girl-friend, who wanted him to marry her daughter. From then on, the wife and the annoyed mother were in constant conflict. One day, the child fell seriously ill and was admitted at the hospital with severe malaria. Despite two weeks of hospital treatment, the child did not recover. The informant decided to ask for advice from a traditional healer (*mganga*). There, she was told that her child was not suffering from malaria, but was bewitched by the mother of her husband's former girl friend. The *mganga* successfully treated the child and protected him from further attacks of the witch.

Dynamics of illness reinterpretation: exclusivity and complementarity

In the study community, *malaria* and witchcraft are two distinct models for understanding illness. The informants stated that witchcraft can never directly cause *malaria*. However, witches are believed to be able to 'play' with the disease. In people's narratives of affliction, the cultural model of *malaria* is linked to the strategies of witches according to two different dynamics of illness reinterpretation. The first we shall call 'exclusivity', the second 'complementarity'.

Exclusivity

The first diagnosis of an illness as 'normal' may be replaced by a new one, where the cause is considered to lie solely in the sphere of spirits or witchcraft. The reason why the models of '*malaria*' and 'witchcraft' are in a exclusive relationship relates to the mode of action of witchcraft which can provoke exactly the same symptoms that people attribute to *malaria*.

The emic explanation of why witches like to imitate *malaria* is that its symptoms easily mislead people, who will attribute them to a common, 'normal' illness that needs hospital treatment. Witchcraft is camouflaged and the witch thereby gains time to destroy the victim . . .

A few informants state that witches can cause a *malaria*-like condition by preparing parasites through magic powers and sending them with the *majini*. These fake parasites cause the same symptoms as *malaria*. Usually, they cannot be detected at the hospital, but even if they can, the treatment with antimalarials fails, because the parasites are not real. According to the interpretation of exclusive explanations, the *mganga* can treat the health problem completely, as it is exclusively provoked by witchcraft. To attend the hospital is only the first step to find out the cause, and as its treatment cannot actually be of any help, there is no need to return to the hospital afterwards.

Complementarity

Exclusivity involves the co-existence and use of alternative causal explanations. Complementarity is used for the situation where multiple causes, interacting with each other, co-exist and *interrelate* when explaining an illness episode. Complementarity is a syncretic mechanism whereby concepts and logic derived from both biomedical and local models are amalgamated in order to give meaning to illness experience.

Anthropologists have applied the idea of different levels of causality to non-western illness aetiologies. The 'immediate' cause makes reference to common aetiologies, such as accidents, infective microorganisms, poison etc. Underlying the 'immediate' cause is the 'ultimate' cause, which is the intentional action of witches, spirits, ancestors or deities. Immediate and ultimate cause are examples of complementarity.

However, this direct relationship between *malaria* and witchcraft was not expressed by the informants in Lipangalala. They explained that an individual who is suffering from spirits or witchcraft can be infected with *malaria*, just like everybody else in the community. *Malaria* and *majini* can simply co-exist, by coincidence, in the same person. People clearly stated that it is not possible for witches to send infected mosquitoes. On the whole, all the accounts indicated that witches can never master living beings stemming from the 'realm of God', but they have the skills to imitate and interfere with them.

That some individuals get *malaria* more often than others is ascribed to their bodily constitution. Bodily strength is considered to be mainly related to innate properties of the person, age and gender. External factors such as weather conditions, hard work or poor nutrition are also perceived to cause body weakness so that the person is more vulnerable to infection. In this sense, witchcraft can also be understood as an indirect, underlying cause of malaria. People reckoned that 'sent spirits' can weaken the bodies of their hosts by feeding on their blood, which renders them more susceptible to any illness, including *malaria*.

Another, more explicit form of complementarity refers to the direct interference of witchcraft with *malaria*. The community is well informed that malaria parasites, injected by mosquitoes, can be detected in the blood and removed with antimalarials. But witches can 'play' with *malaria*. People believe that witches have the skill to make malaria parasites occult in the blood – just as they can make any 'normal' disease occult – in a way that *malaria* cannot be recognized at the hospital.

The health problem is the result of two causes that interact. The spirits sent by witchcraft interfere with 'normal' *malaria*, taking advantage of the disease. In order to eliminate both causes, two types of specialists are needed: first the traditional healer who removes the power of occultation exerted by the sent spirits and afterwards, the medical personnel who treats 'normal' *malaria*.

Antimalarials, majini *and local treatment*
The interdependent and sequential treatment of *malaria* and witchcraft poses significant problems for compliance and adequate treatment with antimalarials. People from the community, and especially the *waganga*, offer elaborate explanations of why the intake of antimalarials before or during the treatment of witchcraft may be inappropriate, ineffective or even dangerous. Antimalarials are felt to be simply inappropriate and useless if the illness is exclusively caused by witchcraft. Moreover, when witchcraft interferes with *malaria*, it is considered ineffective to attend the hospital first, because initially, the *mganga* needs to counteract the spirits' ability to hinder biomedical diagnosis and successful treatment.

Apart from their arts of 'making parasites invisible' and 'imitating *malaria*', *majini* are believed to reject any effective medication, e.g., by forcing the patient to vomit the antimalarials, making his/her skin rigid so that injection needles break, or impeding the penetration of the injection into the blood, resulting in a local abscess. In the worst case, it is said that spirits can induce sudden death after a chloroquine or quinine injection.

A further problem is connected with the combination of antimalarials and local treatment. For healing, the *mganga* uses a selection of herbal remedies, some of which are extremely bitter. Depending on the healer's spirit and on the patient's symptomatology (especially for abdominal pains), there is a tendency to apply 'bitter' *(chungu)* herbs to treat witchcraft. In the local classification of medications, 'bitter' is dichotomically opposed to 'cold' *(baridi)*. Western drugs, too, are included into these two categories. Of interest here is that for 'cold' drugs (e.g. aspirin and paracetamol), there is no need to take precautions of simultaneous intake of different medication, whereas an excess of 'bitter' remedies is considered harmful. To mix the two treatments always requires permission from the *mganga*. As a result of these constraints the risk of non-compliance and delay in attending a biomedical health facility presumably increases.

Although these ideas hardly ever present any problems at the beginning of an illness episode, they can gain relevance during traditional treatment in cases where malaria persists or recurs. Especially for infants and small children who have not yet acquired semi-immunity, a delay of a few days can have lethal consequences.

Treatment of witchcraft usually requires a period of seven days to deactivate the pernicious powers that are 'playing' with *malaria*. In the fight against the spirits *(majini)*, the *mganga* interprets aggravations of the patient's condition as signs of the spirits' rebelliousness. What is interpreted as reactions of the spirits corresponds well, from a biomedical point of view, to the development of inadequately treated or untreated malaria. Although people are aware, too, of the symptomatology of severe malaria, at this stage of the health-seeking process, the hypothesis of witchcraft is strong, precisely because of the previous experience of 'hospital failure'.

Witches are able to imitate malaria and 62% responded that parasites can be made invisible by witchcraft. There is data showing that recurrent malaria episodes (which can be perceived as 'hospital failure') are common in the area as a result of frequent reinfections and high rates of incomplete cures due to resistant parasites. It is also observed that the use of subtherapeutic dosages of antimalarials is often practiced.

Approaches in health information, communication and education have been successful in transmitting knowledge about when and how people should act to receive appropriate and timely treatment for malaria. However, there is little information about treatment failures. This information could effectively be transmitted during the clinical consultation. Rather than discouraging people in their beliefs about witchcraft, the health personnel should thereby play a key role in sensitizing patients and assisting them with clear explanations of prescribed treatment and possible outcomes. The specific recommendations, which could be discussed with the health personnel, are to communicate to people that (i) incomplete treatment can give temporary alleviation, but symptoms might reappear; and (ii) intake of antimalarials prior to hospital attendance (a common practice in the area) can produce partial parasite clearance and thereby explain negative findings from a blood examination. Information about drug resistance should be provided to encourage patients to attend the hospital promptly if symptoms persist or recur.

The challenge is to find out how health personnel can effectively enhance clients' awareness of correct administration of antimalarials and drug resistance. People, including the *waganga*, are certainly open to additional information, provided it makes sense in terms of their own experience.

Now answer the following questions:

1 The people in the study community have a good general understanding of malaria from a biomedical perspective (its cause, symptomatology and treatment), and the use of antimalarials is the first line of treatment. So why are they confronted with ambiguity in the case of actual episodes of malaria? And why do they so easily turn to supernatural explanations? (Remember here earlier discussions of the relationship between beliefs and behaviour, and the concept of *praxis*.)

2 How is syncretism relating to the cause and treatment of malaria expressed in this community? According to Haussman Muela, what effect does this syncretism have on adherence to, and the acceptance of, biomedical treatment? Do you agree with this? If not, why?

↻ Feedback

1 As we have discussed previously, knowledge and beliefs do not necessarily determine behaviour in a direct way, and people tend to be creative and improvise in the often messy situations in which they are confronted with illness. The very nature of malaria, as described by Haussman Muela, adds to this. First, because the symptomatology of malaria itself is inherently ambiguous: its manifestations are variable and its symptoms often diffuse, making a differential diagnosis based on the clinical presentation difficult. Second, because there is widespread acceptance of both biomedical and witchcraft theories, and identical symptomatologies can be equally well explained using either theory. This is exacerbated by the contingencies of actual cases (for example, the child with fever and scratches) and by failures in the biomedical sector.

2 Haussman Muela's informants insisted that witches could not directly cause malaria, but that they could 'interfere' with an episode of malaria. They were well aware that malaria parasites, spread by mosquitoes, could be detected in the blood and removed with antimalarials. But they also thought that witches could make malaria parasites invisible in the blood, so that it would not be recognized in the hospital. Because of this interaction of two causal models, two types of specialist are needed for cure: first the traditional healer who removes the power of the witch, and second biomedics who eliminate the parasites. Haussman Muela uses this syncretic model to explain people's treatment-seeking behaviour for malaria, and to re-examine the issue of adherence, arguing that beliefs in witchcraft and traditional healing (which are often the target of behaviour-change interventions) are not 'cultural obstacles' to the acceptance of biomedical treatment for malaria, but that by offering supernatural explanations for the limitations and failures of biomedicine, they actually reinforce the value of biomedicine in local perceptions.

Summary

The object of medical anthropology is often considered to be ethnomedical systems. Basically, a medical system is a community's ideas and practices relating to illness and health. Anthropologists often describe medical systems as cultural systems – they are culturally constructed and can only be understood in the context of the wider culture of which they are part. Kleinman distinguished three sectors in medical systems: professional, folk and popular. The concept of medical system has been criticized as functionalist; it is too static and implies equilibrium. Medical systems are often discussed in terms of pluralism: the co-existence of different medical traditions or models. Like the concept of medical system itself, the idea of pluralism has also be criticized as being too neat and systematic. In practice different medical traditions and models are often mixed up and used together – syncretism. The point of the critique of medical systems and pluralism is that rather than trying to reveal 'systems' we should focus on studying *practice* (what people actually do when they are ill or suffer misfortune). Health-seeking behaviour is not simply the enactment of 'beliefs' within the confines of a 'culture' or a 'system', but a creative process in which we must recognize the role of invention, innovation, and disorder. The chapter concluded with an excerpt from a paper by Haussman Muela *et al.* in which the concept of syncretism is discussed in detail and illustrated with an ethnographic study of explanations of and treatment-seeking for malaria in Tanzania.

References

Fabian J (1985) Religious pluralism: an ethnographic approach, in Van Binsbergen W and Schoffeleers M (eds) *Theoretical Explorations in the Study of African Religion*. London: Kegan Paul.

Fontaine JL (1998) *Speak of the Devil: Tales of Satanic Abuse in Contemporary England*. Cambridge: Cambridge University Press.

Haussman Muela S, Ribera JM and Tanner M (2000) Fake malaria and hidden parasites – the ambiguity of malaria. *Anthropology and Medicine* 5: 43–61.

Helman CG (1978) 'Feed a cold, starve a fever' – folk models of infection in an English suburban community, and their relation to medical treatment. *Culture, Medicine and Psychiatry* 2: 107–37.

Hobsbawm E and Ranger T (eds) (1983) *The Invention of Tradition*. Cambridge: Cambridge University Press.

Janzen JM (1978) *The Quest for Therapy. Medical Pluralism in Lower Zaire*. Berkeley: University of California Press.

Kleinman A (1980) *Patients and Healers in the Context of Culture*. Berkeley: University of California Press.

Kleinman A (1995) *Writing at the Margin. Discourse between Anthropology and Medicine*. Berkeley: University of California Press.

Last M (1981) The importance of knowing about not knowing. *Social Science and Medicine* 15B: 387–92.

Leslie C (ed) (1976) *Asian Medical Systems*. Berkeley: University of California Press.

Trostle J (1988) Medical compliance as an ideology. *Social Science and Medicine* 27: 1299–308.

5 | Interpreting and explaining sickness

Overview

In their attempts to grapple with the complexity of people's experience of health and sickness, medical anthropologists have developed a number of useful concepts and models. We have already discussed the concept of culture (Chapter 1), which is a more general anthropological concept but one that has been extremely important in medical anthropology, and medical systems and medical syncretism (Chapter 4). In this chapter we will examine a number of other central concepts: the distinction between illness and disease, illness narratives, explanatory models, and different types of aetiology.

Learning objectives

By the end of this chapter you should understand:

- **the distinction between illness and disease and its relevance to understanding how people deal with health and sickness**
- **the idea of explanatory models of sickness, and the criticism of this**
- **the different kinds of aetiology that anthropologists have described and discussed, and the importance of these for contemporary discussions of health and sickness**

Key terms

Aetiology Explanations of the causes of sickness.

Disease Abnormalities in the structure and function of organs and body systems, as defined by biomedicine.

Explanatory model (EM) As used by Arthur Kleinman and many of his followers, an explanatory model consists of the ideas about a particular episode of sickness and its treatment that are employed by all those engaged in the clinical process.

Illness The patient's subjective experience of physical or mental states, whether based on some underlying disease pathology or not.

Illness narrative Stories that patients (but also friends, relatives, healers) tell about sickness. It is often from these stories, collected during long informal discussions with informants, that anthropologists obtain their information about how people experience sickness and suffering.

Kwashiorkor A severe form of protein-energy malnutrition.

> **Sickness** Some medical anthropologists use the term 'sickness' to refer to both illness and disease. Others give 'sickness' a more specialized meaning, using it to refer to the process in which illness and disease are socialized. Here we use the term in the former sense, unless specified.

Illness and disease

Patienthood is a social state and not simply a biological one (Eisenberg and Kleinman 1981). Social and cultural factors are involved in the risk of becoming sick, how sickness is defined and symptoms interpreted, and the response to those symptoms. People *decide* to become (or remain) patients, as well as being *defined and labelled* as patients by doctors.

> Every clinician is familiar with the patient whose disease has been treated successfully but who obstinately persists in complaining of symptoms, as well as the patient who drops out of treatment despite active disease (Eisenberg and Kleinman 1981: 12).

Eisenberg and Kleinman illustrate this with a study that looked at the effectiveness of high-dose antacid therapy for peptic ulcer. All participants in the study were examined with an endoscope at the start of the study and at the end four weeks later. Half the patients received the antacid and the other half a placebo in a double-blind setup. The endoscopic results showed a clear effect of the treatment in the intervention group, but there was no difference in symptoms between the groups: some whose ulcer had healed still had pain and some whose ulcer had not changed no longer had pain (Peterson 1977, cited in Eisenberg and Kleinman 1981: 12).

In order to understand phenomena like this, social scientists developed the distinction between *disease* and *illness* (Eisenberg 1977).

- Doctors diagnose and treat disease – abnormalities in the structure and function of organs and body systems.
- Patients suffer illness – experiences of malfunction in states of being and social function.

Or, as Eric Cassell put it: 'Illness is what the patient feels when he goes to the doctor, disease is what he has on the way home' (Cassell 1976).

Illness and disease may overlap, but are not necessarily coextensive; similar physical pathology can generate different experiences of pain and distress.

Illness is the patient's subjective experience of physical or mental states, whether based on some underlying disease pathology or not. But illness can also be social: the experience of some illnesses is not limited to the symptoms but includes a 'second illness' – the reactions of the social environment, for example the stigma associated with the disorder. Stigmatization is an additional dimension of suffering added to the illness experience (Schulze and Angermeyer 2003). In some cases the social aspect – the stigma – *is* the illness.

Parallel to the distinction between illness and disease, a similar distinction can be made between *cure* and *healing*: doctors may cure disease, but that does not

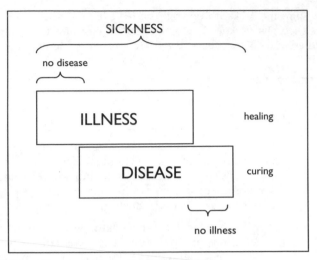

Figure 5.1 Sickness, illness and disease (from Young 1982)

necessarily mean that the patient's illness is healed (Figure 5.1). Cure implies the absence of disease, or its expulsion from the body, whereas healing refers to the improvement of the ailing body and the well being of the ill person. (This will be discussed in more detail in Chapter 10.)

✎ **Activity 5.1**

Go back and re-read the distinction between emic and etic perspectives in anthropology as discussed in Chapter 2. How does this distinction relate to that between illness and disease?

↻ **Feedback**

Regarding the emic/etic distinction, we said that it was often difficult to avoid the impression that etic categories are more real and the etic perspective more true than the emic. This connotation is also present in the illness/disease distinction: because of the general assumption that biomedicine is scientific, and its knowledge therefore more objective, there is a tendency to assume that biomedically defined disease is more real than patient-experienced illness. However, as in the case of emic/etic, illness is no less 'real' than disease.

It is more difficult to invert the illness/disease distinction, as we did with emic/etic, and say that one person's illness is another's disease, however. In the example in Chapter 2 we argued that claiming that the medical view that a child's convulsions are a symptom of severe malaria caused by *plasmodium falciparum* is the etic perspective, and the mother's view that her child has been attacked by spirits is the emic view, could be reversed so that from the mother's perspective, theories of parasites might seem like the doctors culture-bound emic perspective, whereas explanations in terms of spirits, being part of a much wider non-biomedical aetiology, may seem obviously etic. In the case of illness and disease, disease tends to be, by definition, the biomedical perspective (whether viewed as etic or emic), and similarly illness is by definition the subjective experience of the patient.

As with emit and etic, illness cannot always be conveniently separated from disease. While doctors may try to keep their interpretation of disease neutral and objective, subjective aspects of the patient's experience will always impinge, and patients will obviously perceive and experience aspects of the biomedically defined disease as well as the more subjective aspects of the illness.

Illness narratives

Patients order their experience of illness as personal narratives. The illness narrative is a story that the patient tells and significant others retell to give coherence to the distinctive events and long-term course of suffering. The plot, metaphors, rhetorical devices that structure the illness narrative are drawn from more general cultural models, but they are also influenced by personal, individual factors. The narrative does not just reflect the illness experience, but helps to constitute it (Kleinman 1988: 49). We, as researchers, also understand patients' illness experience by creating our own narratives (our ethnographic descriptions of their suffering).

Max's story: an illness narrative

The following example is an abridged version of an illness narrative recorded during an anthropological study of euthanasia in the Netherlands (Pool 2000). Max, a man in his late fifties has been diagnosed with lung cancer and has just completed chemotherapy treatment. In this fragment he talks about his initial diagnosis and treatment. He then goes on to discuss suffering and death.

'I've got a lovely caravan at the seaside. I'd retired, signed off. I'd made my money and I'd had a wonderful year and a half with my wife. We went on holiday, did what we liked. I'd always worked hard, been economical, so we had a good life together. Just the two of us. Kids all married, so no problem. But I was a heavy smoker, I'll be honest with you, and I liked to have a couple of drinks every evening.

'So one day I didn't feel well. There are days like that, aren't there, that you're a bit whingy? So, then I got this terrible pain in my head, here on the right, just above the eyebrow. It was as though my right eye was being pushed out of my head. So I went to see the local doctor. He gave me medicine and said: If it doesn't help, come back. So I phoned him and said: It hasn't helped a bit. So he said: Come and see me immediately and I'll give you something stronger. So he examined me with one of those lights and said: You've probably got sinusitis. So, stronger medicine.

'Then I got another attack of pain in my head. Pressure on the eye. It was terribly painful. So I went to my own GP, Dr Bruijn. I usually have a lung x-ray every year, so I said: Why don't we do the lung x-ray while we're at it? Mr Kraken, he said, you seem to be a bit short of breath as well, so I want to send you for a lung function. So okay, I got a referral and I made an appointment with Dr Schuyt here in the hospital. That was that. I had to come and see him mid-July. We went back to the caravan.

'Two days back at the seaside, I'm having a shave in the morning; I cough up some sputum. Blood! I was shocked. Maybe a burst capillary, my wife said. Then in the evening I coughed up more blood. So I kept an eye on things. Next day, shaving, brushing teeth, you know the routine. More blood! So I phoned the hospital. They said I should come the next day.

'When I arrived Schuyt said: We'll make an x-ray of your lungs and do some blood tests. So, when that'd all been done he said: There's a shadow on your lung. I said: When a doctor tells you there's a shadow on your lung x-ray then in 95 out of 100 cases it's cancer. He said: We'll have to confirm that scientifically first. I said: You're right. He said: We'll have to do a bronchoscopy. I said: Then let's do it.

'And so we did a bronchoscopy on the fifth floor. It wasn't that bad. As long as you do what they tell you. They spray an anaesthetic in your throat and you don't feel a thing. So he was looking and rinsing and pumping and looking again, and I thought: Max, something's wrong, he's seen something.

'On the 28th of June I came back for the results. Schuyt said: Mr Kraken, you have an incurable illness. You've got lung cancer, the small-cell variety. I said: Sounds bad. Because news like that is sobering. I said: What are my chances? He said: Only medicine. I said: What does that imply? He said: Chemotherapy. I said: Okay, so no radiation therapy, no oper-ations? He said: No, only chemotherapy. He said: I've got a proposition. I want to admit you to hospital on the 1st of July. I said: Is it *that* bad? I mean, I'm only a layman, what do I know about those things? No, he said, but it's the holiday season, so we have space. What else could I do but believe him?

'So I came to the hospital on the 1st and for two weeks they did all kinds of tests. And they started the first session of chemotherapy. No problem. I could still walk up and down the passage 40 times. My body was still strong. Second session: also completed with honours. Third session: suddenly a lot weaker. Now I could only walk up and down 12 times before I was tired and had to lie down.

'When I went home after the third session I started to have diarrhoea for the first time. In the meantime I'd also been having radiation therapy, because I'm participating in a scientific trial. I had the first two chemo sessions, then a week of rest, then a week of radiation, then another week of rest. Then came the third chemo session. Then came the diarrhoea, which weakened me even further. Then came the fourth chemo session and I couldn't walk up the corridor even once. I was too weak, get it? But I managed to complete everything. Never gave up. Persevered.

'Then came the fifth session. Monday went perfectly, Wednesday . . . I don't know what's wrong with the Wednesday. Mentally and physically the Wednesday is always the most difficult day. So, next day fever. Today fever. So now we have to wait and see what's going to happen now.

'And then of course there's the mental pressure. You already have the physical burden and then you get a mental burden on top of it. And then a lot depends on your marriage, relationship with the children. How are they coping? As long as nothing goes wrong there are no problems, but as soon as the motor starts failing then there's less understanding. Sometimes they don't want to – or can't – understand that you're sick. Get it?'

'Is it difficult to accept that you're dying?' I asked.

'I accept it. I *have* to accept it, I don't have a choice. I know I've got that illness. I hope I'll be able to extend what's left of my life by doing the chemo and the radiation, that the tumour, those cancer cells, will keep calm. But once they start spreading, then it's just a question of time. Because when they come and say: It's metastasised, then that's the definitive announcement of the end. Do you understand? That would be the end of hope, the future gone.'

'And that acceptance?' I asked. 'When did you realise that? Was it at the start or was it a gradual development?'

'Right from the start. Right from the bronchoscopy. While he was still busy I said to myself: Max, you've got lung cancer. You're going to have to fight to hold onto life a bit longer. I went home – he still had to confirm it on the 28th, but I already knew – and I called the family together. I told them everything. We discussed things and I made my arrangements, right down to the smallest details. The mourning cards have already been addressed. Understand? Financial matters. Insurance, interest, etcetera: it's all been arranged. If I shut my eyes tomorrow, everybody would know exactly what to do. Listen, I manipulated things quite nicely. I managed to arrange very suitable health insurance coverage, for a minimum contribution.'

'How do you see the future now?'

'That's a difficult question, a *very* difficult question. There's a certain . . . how shall I put it . . . fear. Something every cancer patient has. The fear of the moment of truth, the moment you find out it's metastasised. Because you know that, sooner or later, it's going to happen, and you can't do anything about it. And that's terribly difficult, living with that fear. But I just have to live with it because I don't have a choice.

'Have you ever thought about euthanasia?'

'I've discussed it, right at the start, with Dr Schuyt. He made a note in my file. I told him: I don't want to become a Biafran, or someone from Buchenwald or Auschwitz, emaciated, and I don't want to suffer pain. I've always hated pain. I don't like pain. Pain is unnatural. If you've got lung cancer, like me, which isn't painful, then there's no problem. But when you get to the end of the line, like some of the patients here on the ward, then things are different. When I'm like that they have to give me injections so that I don't feel a thing. And when I'm no longer conscious, let them give me an overdose so that I can sleep for all eternity. I've no problem with that. I can't get better anyway. Why should they make me live three weeks longer when I don't even know I'm alive? There's no point. I've discussed all this with my wife and the rest of the family.

'But before they get around to doing that here in this hospital – I mean, you know that – they say: No, first an intravenous drip and a bit of this and a bit of that and some nice tube feeding through your little nose. And before you know it you're lying there, gasping like a fish. And what for, when you're going to die anyway? Why should they extend your suffering like that? Why, when you're going to die any minute anyway, and you've said your goodbyes and everyone supports you and they don't want to see you suffer anymore?

'So, that's what I think about euthanasia. Listen, I know they're messing around with that euthanasia law, and that all kinds of scientists have to write reports. But it's as simple as can be. It's so simple. If you've thought about things, discussed them with your family and GP, you've written everything down, signed it, then who's to prevent you having euthanasia?

They say they're trying to protect you, they want you to hold out, but it's easy to talk when you're healthy. When you're the one in pain, you think differently. So I'm for. Always have been, even before I was sick. If someone with a fine marriage, a happy life, falls sick then you shouldn't force them to suffer. It's not natural. If you have to leave this world, why do it accompanied by pain? Why suffer?'

Max had a short period of remission after the chemotherapy but the cancer soon reappeared and spread. His condition deteriorated rapidly and, when the doctors thought that he had almost reached the end, they increased the dose of morphine, as they had promised him, and he died shortly after.

There are different ways of studying illness narratives. Here we will focus briefly on the plot or narrative structure that emerges from this story, and look at some of the underlying cultural themes.

The plot or narrative structure

On a very basic level, we can identify the following general structure in this story, a structure common to many of the narratives of dying patients in this study.

1 First recognition of symptoms. This leads to recognition and acceptance (in Max's case) or denial.
2 Series of consultations and tests. These cause uncertainty and worry about the exact nature of the illness, the prognosis and the treatment options.
3 The doctor gives the bad news. This leads to crisis, followed by acceptance of the diagnosis, prognosis and recommended treatment (in Max's case) or varying degrees of denial, hope of cure, or acceptance but refusal of treatment.
4 Disclosure (Max) or secrecy (some patients did not even inform their immediate family of their diagnosis).
5 Various stages of treatment, during which the patient either tries to take control or relinquishes this control to the medical staff.
6 Death.

Cultural themes

Underlying this basic narrative are a number of cultural themes taken from wider Dutch society.

Easy death

All the euthanasia requests in the study from which this example has been taken developed against the background of a model of easy death. According to this model, all forms of suffering, pain and physical and mental decline are unacceptable. If the means of avoiding them are available, why suffer unnecessarily when you are going to die shortly anyway? This entails a secular, hedonistic ideology that has banished pain and suffering, and makes no attempt to search for some higher purpose behind suffering. In practice patients shifted the boundary of what was an acceptable level of physical decline, but eventually a limit was often reached and the patient decided that the few remaining pleasures were no longer worth it. In fact, patients often believed in a *right* to die, and that doctors had a concomitant *obligation* to assist. Many patients seemed to think that they were *supposed* to ask for euthanasia if they had cancer. Easy death means less suffering for both patient and relatives, who thereby achieve quick closure. Quite often it was not so much the patient who could not cope with the illness, but the friends and relatives who could no longer take the emotional strain, even after a relatively short illness. On a number of occasions relatives complained: 'How long does this have to last, doctor; can't you speed it up a bit?' Or, in more altruistic terms: 'Can you give him a jab, I don't want him to suffer any longer.'

Control

Patients with terminal illness often wanted to arrange their dying themselves. This was an extreme expression of a key aspect of Dutch culture: the desire to have things under one's own control, formalized in the 'right to self-determination' (*dat regel ik zelf wel*).

Ignorance of this is at the root of the Anglo-American failure to understand Dutch euthanasia. One of the major criticisms of euthanasia in the Netherlands is that euthanasia requests stem from poor pain medication and inadequate terminal care, and that if a patient who requests euthanasia could be transferred to a British hospice, for example, the desire for euthanasia would disappear. This misses the point completely. Not all patients who request euthanasia are in pain and without adequate psychological support; they simply want to choose the moment of death themselves. Euthanasia requests are often long term, a kind of insurance against unnecessary physical decline and loss of control.

Both the plot and the themes are clearly visible in the discourses of many of the cancer patients studied. The themes also emerged clearly in interviews with doctors and relatives as well as in informal discussions in the Netherlands and in the public and media debate on euthanasia.

Explanatory models

People's explanations of the cause of their illness form an important aspect of their illness narratives. In this section and the next we will look at two aspects of people's explanations of illness.

The concept of explanatory models (EMs) was developed by Arthur Kleinman, based on his work in Taiwan, where he found it difficult to reconcile different conflicting, and even contradictory systems of medical beliefs and practices. These covered the whole spectrum from scientific medicine through professional traditional Chinese medicine, sacred and secular forms of folk medicine, and popular 'common sense'.

An explanatory model consists of the ideas about an episode of sickness and its treatment that are employed by all those engaged in the clinical process. Explanatory models are held by both doctors and patients and they guide choices of treatment and give meaning to the experience of sickness. They are anchored in more general explanations of the cause of illness. They are marshalled in response to a particular episode of sickness and are not identical to the general beliefs about sickness in that society (Kleinman 1980: Chapter 3).

In particular they provide explanations for five aspects of illness: cause, when and how symptoms first appeared, the nature of the symptoms, the course of sickness, and treatment. Kleinman distinguishes three dimensions of EMs:

- Lay EMs are idiosyncratic and influenced by personality and local culture; they are only partly conscious and often vague and variable. Practitioner EMs are based on medical theory and scientific logic. They may, however, also include elements of popular culture. For example, Cecil Helman (1978) has shown how ideas from pre-biomedical European medicine are not only central in how patients in England interpret illnesses like the common cold, but infiltrate doctors' explanations as well (Helman 1978).
- Shared and individual EMs. The individual EM that a doctor uses to explain a particular episode of sickness is derived from the theoretical EM that he/she shares with colleagues, and the patient's individual EM is based on the popular explanations of illness shared by the community in general.
- Different editions of individual EMs. Neither doctors nor patients maintain a single unchanging EM throughout the course of an episode of sickness but continually revise their interpretations.

Kleinman describes clinical consultations as transactions between the lay and practitioner EMs for a particular sickness.

Example: explanatory models of kwashiorkor

The idea of explanatory models can be illustrated with an example taken from an anthropological study of kwashiorkor carried out in Cameroon. This case relates to a child brought to the village health centre looking miserable and apathetic, with a big, round, puffy face, and hands, feet and legs so swollen with oedema that the skin was taut and shiny. The child's hair was ginger coloured and soft and silky to the touch.

- **EM1**: The village health worker at the health centre diagnosed the child as having severe protein-energy malnutrition (PEM) caused by a poor diet and he prescribed a protein- and carbohydrate-rich diet.
- **EM2**: The mother said that the child had *ngang* (a term often used to translate 'kwashiorkor' in the vernacular) which was caused by him being followed by twins (twins have special significance in this part of Cameroon, as indeed in much of West Africa). She agreed that diet might also have played a role.
- **EM3**: A local diviner, whom the father had consulted, concluded that the child had *bfaa* (a term also sometimes used as a translation of 'kwashiorkor') which had been caused by some past abomination in the family (such as incest or killing a sacred animal). According to him it had nothing to do with food and could only be cured by carrying out appropriate rituals.
- **EM4**: Nuns at a nearby Catholic hospital became agitated when the case was discussed with them. They became angry that local superstition was being taken seriously and they insisted, based on their outdated knowledge of the bio-medical literature on malnutrition, that the illness was caused by a high-carbohydrate protein-deficient diet. They insisted that the proper remedy was a high-protein diet.
- **EM5**: At the time of this study, researchers working at the Liverpool School of

Tropical Medicine were proposing the hypothesis that kwashiorkor was not caused by a deficient diet but by aflatoxins in the food. They thought that the case supported this hypothesis. *mold on food*

Activity 5.2

How would you relate this example to the distinctions between emic and etic? What would you say are the emic and etic perspectives here?

Feedback

An anthropologist would generally apply an emic analysis to both indigenous and biomedical EMs because both are cultural constructs. That the biomedical perspective is not etic here is emphasized by the fact that there are *three* biomedical EMs. An etic framework would be provided by a theory that encompasses and explains all the EMs involved (a more relativistically inclined anthropologist might argue that no such meta-level is possible and that we are stuck with a series of competing emic perspectives).

Criticism of the EM approach

The EM approach has been, and still is, widely used in medical anthropology and beyond, and is useful for conceptualizing the different interpretations that the patients, their relatives and healers bring to the clinical encounter. It has also been criticized. This criticism focuses on the following issues:

- Like biomedicine, the EM approach focuses on the individual, and as a result the ways in which social relations shape and distribute sickness are ignored.
- This individual focus hides power relationships between groups and classes as a factor in illness. It also ignores the social processes through which behavioural and biological signs are given social meanings.
- It assumes that a patient has only one kind of knowledge about his or her sickness. Patients do not necessarily know their facts in the same way and often give different accounts of the same sickness at the same time. As a result there is no single cognitive model that is the ultimate source of a patient's statements and interpretations (Young 1982).

Alan Young argues that we should take the wider social relations beyond the individual into account when studying sickness, and that there should be more focus on the social conditions of (medical) knowledge production.

Summary

In this chapter we have continued to discuss some of the concepts and models that medical anthropologists have developed in their attempt to understand how people deal with health and sickness. We started with the important distinction between illness and disease. We compared this to the distinction between emic and etic discussed in Chapter 2, and drew attention to some of the problems it entails. We then discussed illness narratives as a way of exploring the patient's experience of illness and the wider cultural models that underlie or give form to that experience. We also discussed the idea of explanatory models, as developed by Arthur Kleinman, and pointed to some of the problems that this very popular concept entails.

References

Cassell EJ (1976) *The Healer's Art: A New Approach to the Doctor–Patient Relationship*. New York: Lippincott.

Eisenberg L (1977) Disease and illness. *Culture, Medicine and Psychiatry* 1: 9–23.

Eisenberg L and Kleinman A (1981) Clinical social science, in Eisenberg L and Kleinman A (eds) *The Relevance of Social Science for Medicine*. Dordrecht: Reidel.

Helman CG (1978) 'Feed a cold, starve a fever' – folk models of infection in an English suburban community, and their relation to medical treatment. *Culture, Medicine and Psychiatry* 2: 107–37.

Kleinman A (1980) *Patients and Healers in the Context of Culture*. Berkeley: University of California Press.

Kleinman A (1988) *The Illness Narratives. Suffering, Healing, and the Human Condition*. New York: Basic Books.

Pool R (2000) *Negotiating a Good Death. Euthanasia in the Netherlands*. New York: The Haworth Press.

Schulze B and Angermeyer MC (2003) Subjective experiences of stigma. A focus group study of schizophrenic patients, their relatives and mental health professionals. *Social Science and Medicine* 56: 299–312.

Young A (1982) The anthropologies of illness and sickness. *Annual Review of Anthropology* 11: 257–85.

6 Situating sickness and health

Overview

This chapter looks in more detail at the context of sickness and focuses on one particular sickness: HIV/AIDS. We start with a discussion of the shift from a focus on individual risk behaviour based on behavioural models derived from social psychology to a broader view of behaviour as culturally determined. This approach is then broadened further by a consideration of political, economic and structural constraints. Through ethnographic case studies we examine the role of power dynamics in particular sexual interactions and the role of 'structural violence' in HIV/AIDS.

Learning objectives

By the end of this chapter you should be able to:

- **discuss the different levels of influences and constraints on the behaviour that puts people at risk of HIV infection**
- **understand the concept of situated risk**
- **have some idea of alternative models of sexual risk behaviour**
- **understand the concept of structural violence**

Key terms

Health belief model A model of health behaviour, very popular in the biomedical and biomedically oriented social science literature, that assumes that behaviour is determined primarily by the 'beliefs' and rational decisions of individuals.

Risk Risk is a term with many diverse but interrelated meanings. According to the *Oxford English Dictionary*, 'risk' is the chance of danger, loss, injury or other adverse consequences. This resembles the popular use of the term. In epidemiology 'risk' refers to the statistical probability of a particular outcome. For example when marriage is described as a risk factor for HIV infection in Africa, it means that statistically women who are married have higher rates of infection than those who are single. This usage has led to the idea of 'risk behaviours', which has in turn led to the identification (and sometimes stigmatization) of risk groups. This problematic aspect of the concept of risk is discussed in detail in the readings below.

Structural violence The constraints on behaviour and options imposed by institutionalized inequalities in wealth and power on those who are underprivileged: mainly women, the poor, those of colour.

From individual behaviours to cultural context

'Risk', already a central concept in epidemiology and a topic that had received significant anthropological and sociological attention, suddenly took on a new significance with the advent of HIV/AIDS. Medical research programmes became acutely interested in 'risky behaviours' that were assumed to be contributing to the spread of HIV and 'risk groups' that were thought to be the source of infection in communities (prostitutes and truck drivers, for example).

Most of the social science research on HIV, especially in the early years of the epidemic, focused on the behaviour of individuals and took the form of Knowledge, Attitudes, Behaviour and Practices (KABP) surveys. Much of what was referred to as anthropological research in these settings was basically the use of qualitative methods such as open interviews and focus group discussions – often in the form of short 'rapid appraisals' (see the criticism of defining anthropology in terms of qualitative methodology in Chapter 1). This research was aimed at collecting quantitative data on frequencies of sexual practices and on understanding the largely individual reasons and motivations for this behaviour. It was intended to contribute to the development and implementation of interventions to change individually based risk behaviour.

However, anthropological and sociological research on sexual behaviour and risk in the context of HIV/AIDS has managed to shift the focus from individual behaviours to the wider social and cultural settings in which that behaviour is embedded, and to the cultural models and meanings that organize it. Attention has been given to the local, emic cultural concepts and systems of classification through which people define and construct sexual experience in an attempt to move away from the etic concepts of biomedicine. It has become clear, as Parker has argued, that many of the key categories used in biomedicine to describe sexual behaviour or account for the vectors of infection are not relevant in all cultural contexts. He gives 'homosexuality' and 'prostitution' as examples (Parker 2001).

Activity 6.1

1   Can you think of other categories or classifications that are commonly used in biomedically oriented HIV/AIDS related research on sexual behaviour? What are the potential consequences of using these uncritically in different cultural settings with which you are familiar?
2   Parker states that 'new knowledge and information about perceived sexual risk will always be interpreted within the context of pre-existing systems of meaning'. Think of an example (preferably from your own experience) of information that has been provided to a community as part of a health intervention but that has been interpreted completely differently to how it was intended.

Feedback

1 Almost all the central concepts involved in studying sexual behaviour in Africa are ambiguous: marriage, spouse, regular partner, casual partner, partner reduction, risk, change, promiscuity, monogamy, faithfulness, abstinence and so forth. It is impossible, for example, to draw any clear line between 'casual' and 'regular' partners (two categories used uncritically in most sexual behaviour surveys and qualitative studies in Africa) in a particular cultural setting, never mind making comparisons across the continent. Or take the term 'marriage'. Among the Baganda in Uganda, 'marriage' can be civil, religious, or customary, or the couple might simply cohabit and refer to this as marriage. Depending on how they were married and the woman's position in the man's sequence of partners, she may also be called *omukyala oweka* (the wife for the home), *mukyala mukulu* (elder wife), *mukyala owempetta* (wife who bears my ring), *mukyala siniya* (senior wife), *mukyala namba emu* (wife number one) or *maama wa baana* (mother of my children) (Nyanzi et al. 2004). These would all end up as 'wife' or 'spouse' in questionnaires. 'Behaviour change' is another term. What is meant may vary from radical partner reduction or regular condom use to having once experimented with a condom. 'Partner reduction' is particularly problematic. When people say they have reduced the number of partners in sexual behaviour change surveys, what do they mean? They are ostensibly talking about numbers, but these cannot be measured in any meaningful way. And 'reduction' might simply mean that they have avoided potential sexual encounters that they think they might not have avoided in the past. These ambiguous meanings have serious consequences for the usefulness of the data collected in comparisons between areas with different categorizations, and for the interventions based on those data.

2 In a study in Uganda, for example, it was found that condom use, promoted for years as something positive – a means of preventing HIV infection – was underreported because of its negative connotations – a sign of promiscuity implying the spread of HIV (Pool et al. 2005). In fact, throughout Africa, condoms are associated with casual sex and as a result people are reluctant to use them in relationships that are defined as stable (but in which women are at most risk).

Situated risk

Anthropological research on HIV/AIDS has moved from a narrow focus on individual behaviour to a broader consideration of the cultural setting in which this behaviour takes place. It has also made it clear that many of the theoretical models of behaviour, taken uncritically from social psychology, which focus on the individual and assume a rational basis for decision making, are inadequate. In this section we will consider in more detail one ethnographic study by Bloor et al. (1993) that focuses on the micro-social context of the sexual encounter in order to explain the variability of risk behaviour among male prostitutes in Glasgow by offering an alternative explanatory framework.

HIV-related risk practices among Glasgow male prostitutes: reframing concepts of risk behavior

Defining unsafe sex as the practice of anogenital intercourse, this article focuses on comparisons between that minority of Glasgow male prostitutes who reported currently practicing unsafe commercial sex and their fellows who reported always currently practicing safer commercial sex.

Aspects of risk behavior in commercial sex

Ten of the 32 respondents reported that they were currently engaging in at least occasional anogenital sex with 'punters' (clients). Sixteen respondents reported currently engaging only in safer (nonanal) commercial sex. We have no information on the sexual practices of six subjects. It will be demonstrated that a distinction between those undertaking unsafe and safer sex can be made in respect to the exercise of power in the prostitute-client encounter. Those prostitutes undertaking unsafe commercial sex were constrained to do so by client control.

This variation in practice among those practicing unsafe sex was mirrored by a similar variation in their biographical circumstances. Participants included a nonstreetworker, as well as streetworkers, those who were identified as being gay and those who were not, those who were injecting drug users and those who were not, those who were novice prostitutes and those who were not. This is not to argue that there is no association between, for example, several years' experience as a prostitute and the practice of safer commercial sex. But experience is neither a necessary nor a sufficient condition for safer sex, because there were both novice prostitutes who were practicing safer sex and experienced prostitutes who were practicing unsafe sex.

An absolute distinction between those currently practicing safer sex and those currently practicing unsafe sex cannot be made on the basis of the prostitutes' biographical circumstances. The research literature on risk behavior, in any case, lays more stress on the subject's perceptions and psychological state than on his biographical circumstances. A series of studies of HIV-related risk behavior has conceived of risk-taking as a volitional act arising out of a sense of personal invulnerability. The subject knows how the virus is transmitted but believes that his personal chance of becoming infected is slight.

Only one of the present sample, however, could be represented as voluntarily engaging in anal sex in this way without concern for possible HIV infection. The other respondents appear to be engaging in unsafe commercial sex *despite* a concern with HIV transmission, despite a perceived susceptibility to infection. Traditionally this kind of apparent inconsistency has been treated as an instance of the well-known disjunction between attitudes and behavior. Instead, our approach will be to treat this disjunction as constrained by the strategic relationship between prostitute and punter, as a function of client control of the sexual encounter. It will be argued that the remaining subjects who engaged in unsafe commercial sex did so because they were unable to contest the client's control of the encounter; unsafe sex is a consequence of particular kinds of strategic relations, not prostitutes' health beliefs. This requires an ethnographic understanding of the immediate circumstances of the commercial sex act.

Variations in prostitute-client power relations

There is considerable variation in the verbal and nonverbal exchanges that preface male prostitute-client sexual encounters. Some of our respondents took immediate directive control of the encounter, openly negotiating with clients over the type of sex to be performed, price, and location. Others behaved much more passively, even to the extent, in some cases, of failing to make it clear in advance that they were expecting payment. It will be shown that the preface to the encounter shapes the encounter itself. Those prostitutes who failed to seize directive control of the encounter could find themselves subject to client control, with safer or unsafe sex at the client's discretion.

Male prostitution is a stigmatized and illegal activity, and street prostitution takes place in public settings. Circumspect approaches to potential clients are readily understandable. The most common approach was the cautious nonverbal eye contact known as 'cottaging'. Only one of the streetworking respondents was seen to address punters openly without reserve and circumspection.

The point to be emphasized is that where encounters were covert and largely silent, they were characterized by a high degree of ambiguity and were thus wide open to misunderstandings. The furtive and largely nonverbal exchanges that typically precede the sex act may embrace little or no discussion about either price or the kind of sexual services being offered. Indeed, it may even be ambiguous to the punter that this is a commercial transaction at all. The majority of the 32 prostitutes self-reported as gay (ten self-reported as 'straight' and two as 'bisexual') and the majority of these reported that they sometimes went cruising as well as 'renting' (prostituting). All the sites where the prostitutes worked were also cruising or cottaging sites and gay cruisers constituted most of the traffic. Moreover, at least one prostitute told us that he felt unable to broach the topic of money directly.

Under these circumstances, it is hardly surprising that disputes about money were frequently reported. Punters would dispute that any money at all was involved and reject the prostitute's claims as attempted extortion. Alternatively, the punter might recognize that this was a commercial transaction but after the event might dispute the fee, particularly because there was no standard rate for male prostitutes' services (itself a reflection of covert and ambiguous prostitute-client relations), with the prostitutes charging what the market would bear.

Violence was a frequent feature of streetwork. By no means all of it was associated with disputes about payment. One of our respondents was alleged to be attracting punters with the object of 'rolling' (mugging) them and two others reported that they had started their careers by rolling clients before graduating to prostitution proper. During the fieldwork period, three subjects were charged with assault and a fourth was imprisoned on assault charges.

If there is often a dangerous ambiguity surrounding the all-important topic of payment, then it seems clear that a similar ambiguity may also surround the topic of the kind of sexual services being provided. Beyond the world of prostitution, ambiguity and sex are strongly associated. This may have been behind the contention of one of the four nonstreetworkers, who had 'graduated' from streetwork, that those streetworkers he knew were 'inarticulate' and unable to negotiate with clients. On a few occasions we encountered embarrassed reactions from respondents as we asked them questions about their work. Such reactions were, however, atypical even among novice female prostitutes. The experienced nonstreetworker's comment about inarticulateness refers not to a tongue-tied reticence but rather to a failure to seize the interactional initiative, to a lack of the social skills to cut through the silence, clear up the ambiguity, and state what services they are willing to provide at what price.

Yet not all streetworkers lacked these social skills. Four respondents would ask punters for the money up front, and a fifth respondent would ask the punter to show him the money first. Getting the money up front was the universal practice among the female street-workers. This practice has the obvious advantage that the punter is unable to enforce compliance and ensure dominance by threatening to withhold payment. In addition, the demand for prior payment helps to dispel any ambiguity over whether or not this is a commercial transaction and (more important still) it provides an occasion for open discussion about what kinds of sexual services are being offered and at what price.

For male prostitutes, to demand payment up front contravened customary practice. Nevertheless, those subjects who were demanding the money up front reported that it was a successful strategy.

To seize the interactional initiative ('I'm sorry but I charge') or to demand advance payment ('No money, no deal') is to exercise a strategy of influence. Power, according to Foucault, is no commodity or attribute of status, but a strategic relationship. Power is inherent within a relationship, but dominance – manifested and felt imbalances and inequalities in that strategic relationship – varies. In the absence of countervailing strategies from the prostitute it seems that the client is the dominant party.

This is the pivotal point. For our 'unsafe' subjects, it did not matter that they were concerned about HIV infection, because the client, not the prostitute, was in control: type of sex was a matter for the client's discretion.

What distinguishes our 'unsafe' prostitutes from those practicing safer sex is that the former lacked those countervailing techniques of power. Safer sex is thus associated with countervailing prostitute strategies of power that wrest domination of the encounter from the client. Some of these strategies have already been noted and rely for their effectiveness on making explicit the hidden agenda of the encounter, stripping away the ambiguity to allow overt discussions of services and prices. An alternative prostitute strategy is the attempt to screen out clients who seek anal penetration. This is best achieved either by building up a 'book' of regular clients, or else by securing a 'sugar daddy' who will provide most of the prostitute's needs, which may be supplemented by extras provided by a few 'regulars.'

One final point is that none of these countervailing techniques – demanding the money up front, opening up the hidden agenda, confining oneself to regular known clients – is a sure defence against all vagaries of fortune.

Paradoxically, in view of our previous assertion of the relationship between ambiguity, violence, and unsafe sex, attempts to contest client control may themselves, on occasion, lead to violence.

Models of risk behavior

Our view of risk behavior as being largely shaped by the immediate situation of the sexual encounter is a rather different approach from psychosocial models of risk behavior, such as the 'health belief' model, that seek to explain health behavior by reference to individual perceptions (for example, of vulnerability, of severity of health threat). In the field of illness behavior, these psychosocial models were quickly contested by authors who stressed the structural and cultural causes of variations in the use of health services; they proposed collectivity-oriented models of illness behavior in opposition to the individualized models.

A social-structural model of risk behavior seems, however, like the health belief model, of limited application to commercial homosexual encounters. As previously stated, social, structural, and cultural variables, such as streetworker or nonstreetworker, gay or straight, experienced or novice, produced neither the necessary nor the sufficient conditions for safer commercial sex.

Nevertheless, the limited applicability of both approaches (psychosocial and structural-cultural) should not blind us to the fact that each approach has resonances with some of the data on risk practices presented earlier. There is, in principle, a third model option according to which the range of activities subsumable under illness behavior (perception of symptoms, interpretation, the search for an appropriate remedy) might be conceptualized by reference to Schutz's work on 'systems of relevance.'

The systems of relevance are essentially a conceptual scheme for a social theory of cognition. 'Topical' relevances determine whether an object (e.g., a health threat) is perceived. 'Motivational' relevances determine whether and how far an object is investigated (the subject's degree of concern about the possible health threat).

'Interpretational' relevances determine how an object is investigated and interpreted (is it or is it not a health threat?). Each of these sets of relevances may be 'intrinsic' (that is, volitional) or 'imposed' (that is, constrained). Associated with given interpretations are 'recipes for action,' culturally specific and culturally prescribed procedures for acting toward an interpreted object to bring forth desired results. In other words, associated with a given health threat (e.g., unsafe sex) there may be a particular remedy (e.g., getting the money beforehand).

The model is heuristic rather than predictive, but has certain advantages. First, the scheme incorporates both volition and constraint, since relevances may be either 'intrinsic' or 'imposed.' Thus, in the case of commercial homosexual sex, unsafe sex arises primarily out of *imposed* motivational relevances.

Second, the scheme links perception and action in the association between interpretation and recipe. Thus, in the present case, safer commercial sex is associated with certain recipes that seize the interactional initiative for the prostitute. Third, stress is laid on the culturally acquired and culturally specific character of both interpretations and recipes for action. Thus, successful recipes for safer sex may be learned and passed on. Fourth, it gives importance to immediate contextual factors as precursors for behavior. This is so not only because the immediate context provides the initial stimulus to interpretation and action, but also because the topical relevance of a given object is always provisional and liable to disruption and supercession by other immediate contextual factors in the individual's perceptual field: risk behavior is treated as an emergent and situated product.

✎ Activity 6.2

1　What is the main point that the authors make in this paper?
2　How did male prostitutes change the power relationship with clients and avoid unsafe sex?
3　What is the authors' main criticism of the health belief model?
4　Popular explanations of health behaviour in the media often rely on assumptions similar to those employed in the health belief model. Think of a recent example of a public or media discussion of health-related behaviour that was based (if only implicitly) on the assumptions of the health belief model.

C♪ **Feedback**

1 Bloor *et al.* show how risk was related to the unequal power relationship between prostitute and client, resulting from the covertness and the ambiguity of the interaction and the greater age of the client. Unsafe sex was associated with client control over the encounter, whereas safer sex was associated with the prostitute taking control of the interaction. They show that unsafe commercial sex, in this setting, was not a matter of volition based on misconceptions about the degree of risk (most of the prostitutes were acutely aware of the risks) – beliefs – but on the power dynamics of the situation.

2 By demanding money up front, for example, the prostitutes could dispel the ambiguity of the situation by seizing the interactional initiative. This put them in control of the encounter and made it easier to refuse unsafe sex.

3 The main criticism of the health belief model is that health behaviours are not determined primarily by the 'beliefs' and the rational decisions of individuals, but are determined, or at least constrained, by the power dynamics of the situation.

4 During the past few years there has been a widely publicized reluctance by parents in the UK to accept their children receiving the triple MMR (measles, mumps, rubella) vaccination. This reluctance is said to be based on the popular acceptance of the results of a controversial theory – which has since been disproved – that MMR is linked to autism. It is generally assumed – though not often explicitly stated – that this reluctance stems from parents' 'belief' that the MMR jab increases the risk of autism, and that they obtained this 'wrong belief' from media coverage of the earlier study.

Structural violence

In the reading above we have seen how individual risk is dependent on the power dynamics of specific interactional situations. But a much broader array of political, economic, historical and structural factors (poverty, exploitation, gender inequality, racism, discrimination) may also play a central role in influencing and constraining behaviour and creating vulnerability. This has been referred to as 'structural violence'. In the next abridged reading Paul Farmer (1997) combines detailed ethnography with an analysis of the wider context of structural violence in order to understand HIV/AIDS in Haiti.

Ethnography, social analysis, and the prevention of sexually transmitted HIV infection among poor women in Haiti

Social scientists and physicians alike have long known that the socioeconomically disadvantaged have higher rates of disease than do those not hampered by such constraints. But by what mechanisms and processes might social factors be transformed into personal risk? How do forces as disparate as sexism, poverty, and political violence become embodied as individual pathology? As HIV advances, it is becoming clear that, in spite of a great deal of epidemiological and ethnographic research, we do not yet understand risk and how it is structured.

Recent trends in the pandemic should undermine the falsely reassuring – and inappropriately stigmatizing – notion of discrete 'risk groups' to be identified by epidemiologists.

Increasing incidence of HIV disease among women is a case in point. The United Nations (UNDP 1992) observed that, 'for most women, the major risk factor for HIV infection is being married.' It is not marriage, however, that places women at risk. Throughout the world, most women with HIV infection are living in poverty. The study of the dynamics of HIV infection among poor women affords a means of examining the complex relationships between power, gender, and sexuality.

Although many observers would agree that forces such as these are the strongest enhancers of risk for infection, this subject has been neglected in both the biomedical and anthropological literature on HIV disease to the benefit of a narrowly behavioral and individualistic conception of 'risk.'

Why might this be so? Most epidemiological and biomedical journals do not consider racism, sexism, and class differentials to be subjects of polite discussion. But significant theoretical and methodological difficulties also impede investigation of these issues (as does, perhaps, a sense of helplessness about the practical implications of careful examination of such issues). Some of these difficulties are perennial: how broadly must the net be cast if we are to capture both the large-scale forces structuring risk and the precise mechanisms by which these forces affect the lives of individuals?

I would like to examine the relationship between poverty, gender, and HIV disease by presenting data from Haiti. I present these data by telling one woman's story, and then continue by discussing a study of HIV infection among poor women from rural Haiti. In so doing, one moves from biography to the structural violence that to no small extent shapes biography by constraining options available to women living in poverty.

HIV, gender, poverty: Guylene's story

Guylene Adrien was born in a dusty village in the middle of Haiti's infertile central plateau. Like other families, the Adriens were poor. Guylene was the third of four children, a small family by Haitian standards. It was to become smaller still: Guylene's younger sister died in adolescence of cerebral malaria. Guylene's oldest sister, embittered by the loss of all four of her children, eventually left for the Dominican Republic, where she works as a servant. When Guylene was 14 or 15 a family acquaintance, Occident Dorzin, made it clear to Guylene that he was attracted to her. 'But he was already married, and I was a child. When he placed his hand on my arm, I slapped him and swore at him and hid in the garden.'

Dorzin approached Guylene's father to ask for her hand in plasaj (a potentially stable sexual union widespread in rural Haiti). Before she was 16, Guylene moved, with a man 20 years her senior, to a village about an hour away from her parents. She was soon pregnant. Occident's wife was not pleased, and friction eventually led to dissolution of the newer union. In the interim, however, Guylene gave birth to two children.

Guylene and her nursing son returned to her parent's house. She then met a young man named Osner, and set off to try conjugal life a second time. The subsequent months were difficult ones. Guylene's father died later that year, and her son, cared for largely by her sister, was often ill. Guylene was already pregnant with her third child, and she and Osner lacked almost everything that might have made their new life together easier. After the baby was born, in 1985, they decided to move to the city.

Osner and Guylene spent almost three years in the city. These were hardscrabble times. Political violence was resurgent, especially in the slum areas. The couple was often short of work.

In 1987, three 'unhappy occurrences' came to pass. A neighbor was shot, fatally, during one of the military's regular night time incursions into the slum. A few weeks later, Guylene received word that her son had died 'abruptly.' And, finally, Osner became gravely ill. It started, Guylene recalled, with weight loss and a persistent cough. He returned to Do Kay a number of times in the course of his illness.

Osner reported a lifetime total of seven sexual partners, including Guylene. At his death in September 1988, it was widely believed, in the Kay area, that he had died from the new disease; his physicians concurred.

By early June, Guylene was ill: she had lost weight, had amenorrhea, and felt short of breath on exertion. But it was her child's symptoms – abdominal pain, irritability, poor food intake – that brought her, on June 18, 1992, to the clinic. After reviewing Osner's chart, the physician suggested that she be tested for HIV, and she was informed of her positive serology.

In mid-November Guylene responded to the advances of a soldier. Because Guylene's physicians had gone to some trouble to prevent her from having unprotected sexual intercourse, we were anxious to know how our conversations about this subject may have figured in her decision – if decision is the term – to conceive another child. But she was impatient with questions, tired of talking about sadness and death: 'Will the baby be sick? Sure he could be sick. People are never not sick. I'm sick . . . he might be sick too. It's in God's hands. I don't know.'

Currently, Guylene draws to the close of her fifth pregnancy, which may well culminate in another death. Two other children are dead; two others have long looked to a father or grandmother for the bulk of their parenting. Guylene's own sisters are dead, missing, or beaten into submission by the hardness of Haiti. Few of her nephews and nieces have survived to adulthood.

Linking micro to macro

When compared to age-matched North Americans with AIDS, Guylene, like other rural Haitians with AIDS, has a sparse sexual history. In fact, there is little about Guylene's story that is unique; it is recounted in some detail because it brings into relief many of the forces that effectively constrained not only her options, but those of most Haitian women.

Such, in any case, is my opinion after caring for dozens of poor women with HIV disease. There is a deadly monotony in their stories: young women – or teenaged girls – driven to Port-au-Prince by the lure of an escape from the harshest poverty; once in the city, each worked as a domestic; none managed to find the financial security so elusive in the countryside. The women I interviewed were straightforward about the non-voluntary aspect of their sexual activity: In their opinions, they had been driven into unfavorable unions by poverty. Over the past several years, the medical staff of the clinic on Do Kay has diagnosed dozens of cases of HIV infection in people presenting to the clinic with a broad range of complaints. With surprisingly few exceptions, however, those so diagnosed shared a number of risk factors, as a small-scale case–control study suggests (Table 6.1). The study was conducted by interviewing the first 17 women diagnosed with symptomatic HIV infection who were residents of Do Kay or its two neighboring villages.

Their responses to questions posed during the course of a series of open-ended interviews were compared with those of 17 age-matched, seronegative controls. In both groups, ages ranged from 17 to 37, with a mean of about 25 years. None of these 34 women had a history of prostitution; none had used illicit drugs; only one, a member of the control group,

Table 6.1 Case–control study of HIV infection in 34 rural Haitian women

Patient characteristics	HIV disease (N 17)	Control (N 17)
Number of sexual partners	2.7	2.2
Partner of truckdriver	9	1
Partner of soldier	7	0
Partner of peasant only	0	15
Port-au-Prince residence	14	4
Worked as servant	11	0
Years of education	4.8	4
Received blood transfusion	0	1
Used illicit drugs	0	0
Received > 10 IM injections	11	13

had a history of transfusion. None of the women in either group had more than six sexual partners. In fact, four of the afflicted women had had only one sexual partner. Although women in the study group had (on average) more sexual partners than controls, the difference is not striking. Similarly, there was no clear difference between the study and control group vis-à-vis the number of intramuscular injections received or years of education.

The chief risk factors in this small study group seemed to involve not the number of partners in a lifetime, but rather the professions of these partners. Fully 14 of the women with HIV disease had histories of sexual contact with soldiers or truckdrivers. Histories of extended residence in Port-au-Prince and work as a domestic were also strongly associated with a diagnosis of HIV disease.

Conjugal unions with salaried soldiers and truckdrivers who are paid on a daily basis reflect these women's quest for economic security. In this manner, truckdrivers and soldiers have served as a 'bridge' to the rural population, just as North American tourists seem to have served as a bridge to the urban Haitian population. Once introduced into a sexually active population, HIV will work its way into those with no history of residence in the city, no history of contact with soldiers or truckdrivers, and no history of work as a domestic. The research presented here underlines the importance of social inequalities of the most casual, everyday sort in determining who is most at risk for HIV infection.

When ethnographic and clinical-epidemiological research are linked to unflinching social analysis, the contours of a rapidly changing epidemic – and the forces promoting HIV transmission – come into focus. Concluding that, in Haiti, 'poverty and economic inequity serve as the most virulent co-factors in the spread of this disease' it is possible to identify seven other socially conditioned forces enhancing rates of HIV transmission among Haitian women. These include:

1 gender inequality, especially concerning control of land and other resources;
2 traditional patterns of sexual union, such as *plasaj*;
3 emerging patterns of sexual union, such as the serial monogamy described by Guylene and by most of our patients (many of whom implicate poverty in the undermining of these unions);
4 prevalence of STDs and other genital-tract infections and perhaps more significantly, lack of access to treatment for them;
5 lack of timely response by public-health authorities, a delay related not merely to lack of resources but the persistence of a political crisis;

6   lack of culturally appropriate prevention tools;

7   political violence, much of it state-sponsored and directed at poor people.

Each of these factors and forces was relevant in Guylene's experience, and they are relevant in the lives of most of our patients. These are the 'givens,' the structural violence of their country and, indeed of the larger historical system in which it is ensnared.

These are not factors regularly discussed in the medical journals. Yet there is ample reason to believe that similar factors help to determine the epidemiology of HIV infection in wealthier countries too, especially those characterized by high indices of economic disparity, such as the United States.

One reason social forces are not candidly discussed in the biomedical press may be related to the way AIDS research funds have been doled out. Quick to associate anthropology with studies of exotic animal sacrifice, say, or ritual scarification, those in control of funds ask anthropologists to perform 'rapid ethnographic assessments' of settings with high rates of HIV transmission.

In my view, obscuring 'the totality of the larger society's structure' (including its place in international systems) is all too often the mission of anthropological assessment when the goal of such assessment is to assign origins or vectors for disease in such 'barbaric' practices as animal sacrifice and blood ritual. In the vast majority of settings in which anthropologists work, HIV is transmitted through much more mundane mechanisms.

Finally, such 'exotic' practices are out of the ordinary, isolated and to a large extent voluntary. By associating them with AIDS, do we not silently reassure ourselves that the disease we study is equally voluntary, exceptional, and experience-distant? If that is the profile of medial anthropology in the AIDS pandemic, Haiti has a lesson to teach it.

✎ Activity 6.3

1   What is 'structural violence'? Make a note of the main characteristics.

2   How does Farmer relate the analysis of wider structural issues to the ethnographic study of specific situations and cases?

3   Think about another infectious disease that you are familiar with. What role do you think the various social forces that Farmer discusses – economic pressure, patterns of sexual union, gender inequality, cultural factors, politics, concurrent disease, access to medical services – play in the distribution of this disease? What is the contribution of individual behaviour and agency? Write a short description of how these factors are linked and illustrate this with a diagram.

↻ Feedback

1   Structural violence basically refers to the effects of institutionalized inequalities in wealth and power on those who are underprivileged: mainly women, the poor, those of colour. Farmer argues that we need to look not just at disease and individual risk, but also at its links with the wider context of poverty, sexism, racism – structural violence – in order to understand the unequal distribution of disease. He argues that we do not yet have an adequate understanding of this because structural violence is not considered the subject of 'polite discussion' in the medical and epidemiological journals,

and because both the epidemiological and anthropological literature have adopted a narrow behavioural and individual conception of risk.

2 In arguing for a broader approach that takes macro-social forces into account, Farmer does not neglect a micro-level focus on the ethnographic detail of individual biography, agency and local cultural context: 'Many of the issues of individual agency are illuminated by examining the gritty details of biography; life histories must be embedded in ethnography if their representativeness is to be understood. These local understandings are to be embedded, in turn, in the larger-scale historical system of which the fieldwork site is part . . . Only through such a broad approach will the role of "structural violence" come into view' (Farmer 1997:416).

Summary

This chapter examined some of the very extensive anthropological literature on HIV/AIDS. We presented criticism of the simplistic assumption – in much of the biomedical and biomedically oriented social science literature – that risk behaviour is determined by individuals making rational decisions and choices (based on the health belief model). We presented Bloor *et al.*'s ethnographic study of male prostitutes in Glasgow to show how individual risk behaviour can be influenced by micro-level power dynamics. We then went on to discuss the wider issues of structural violence as presented in the work of Paul Farmer in Haiti.

References

Bloor MJ, Barnard MA, Finlay A and McKeganey NP (1993) HIV-related risk practices among Glasgow male prostitutes: reframing concepts of risk behavior. *Medical Anthropology Quarterly* 7: 152–69.

Farmer P (1997) Ethnography, social analysis, and the prevention of sexually transmitted HIV infection among poor women in Haiti, in Inhorn M and Brown P (eds) *The Anthropology of Infectious Disease*. Amsterdam: Gordon and Breach.

Nyanzi S, Nyanzi B, Kalina B and Pool R (2004) Mobility, sexual networks and exchange among bodabodamen in southwest Uganda. *Culture, Health and Sexuality* 6: 23–54.

Parker R (2001) Sexuality, culture, and power in HIV/AIDS research. *Annual Review of Anthropology* 30: 163–79.

Pool R, Kamali A and Whitworth J (2005) Understanding sexual behaviour change in southwest Uganda, *AIDS Care*.

UNDP (1992) *Young Women: Silence, Susceptibility, and the HIV Epidemic*. New York: UNDP.

7 The relationship between anthropology and biomedicine

Overview

As we discussed earlier, the main reason why medical researchers and public health professionals are interested in collaborating with anthropologists is because anthropologists are thought to have knowledge of – or the tools to find out about – local culture. We have argued in the first two chapters that this is only one aspect of anthropology. In Chapter 2 we argued that studying the *Other* gave anthropology a critical perspective on what is accepted as normal, obvious, common sense. Given this approach, it seems logical that anthropologists would not automatically accept the widespread assumption (particularly in the West) that biomedicine is qualitatively different from other medical systems – that it is superior because it is objective and scientific and more effective in really curing disease. The crucial question then is: how should anthropology relate to biomedicine? If biomedicine is simply one of many ethnomedicines, all equally valid, then how can anthropologists collaborate in the wider biomedical project of research and intervention? If anthropologists accept that biomedicine is unique – more objective and culturally neutral – than other medicines, then on what basis can anthropology privilege biomedicine and raise it above critical scrutiny? In this chapter, building on the distinction between anthropology of/in medicine, we will suggest some answers to these questions. First we will argue that biomedicine is itself a cultural system – that it is not privileged above other cultural systems. We will then consider a number of options for the interaction between anthropology and biomedicine.

Learning objectives

After working through this chapter, you will be better able to:

- outline the different ways in which medical anthropology relates to biomedicine
- critically evaluate the assumption that biomedicine's categories and priorities are given rather than socially and culturally contingent
- give examples of how to situate biomedicine as a cultural product

Key terms

Bracketing Setting on hold, or excluding from consideration, certain concepts or aspects of a situation; for example studying a patient's experience of an illness while ignoring (though aware of) the biological disease.

Materialism The theory that everything that really exists is material, and that mental states or consciousness are merely derived from material substance.

Mystification A process by which the nature of reality is hidden in such a way that it serves to maintain the status quo and protect those in power from criticism.

Reductionism The notion that complex phenomena can be explained by reducing them to some more basic level; for example the idea that disease is basically the physical malfunctioning of organs and cells.

Biomedicine as a cultural system

Western science (and biomedicine) has its roots in the distinction, derived from ancient Greek philosophy, between reality and appearance. A well-known example from the book *The Republic* by the ancient Greek philosopher Plato, has a group of people chained in a cave with their backs to the light. All they have ever seen is the shadows of people passing by outside the cave. What they see is only an appearance, an illusion. It takes someone to escape from the chains and venture outside the cave to discover the true, underlying reality. There is a long Western tradition that assumes that behind the changing and often chaotic surface of events there is a more fundamental, permanent, universal reality (whether God's grand plan or scientific truth). Paul Unschuld, the historian of Chinese medicine, has claimed that monotheism (the belief in a single all-powerful god) has had an important influence on biomedicine, legitimizing the idea of a single, underlying truth and fostering intolerance toward alternative paradigms (Kleinman 1995: 27).

Western science is *materialist*; it assumes that reality is basically material, that nature is physical and we can obtain objective knowledge of it independently from our senses and the methods and instruments used to observe it. This leads to a reductionist view of sickness: it is confined to individual physical bodies rather than being a social phenomenon situated in groups, it is reducible to the malfunctioning of the basic material building blocks – cells and molecules – rather than disrupted social relations, its signs are visible under the microscope or in the test tube rather than in the complaints and stories of the sufferer, and cure is in the form of a pharmaceutical magic bullet rather than healing.

Rather than working within (or under) biomedicine and accepting natural science and biomedical categories and priorities as given, anthropologists can distance themselves from biomedicine (and science) and study it as a cultural phenomenon, as one form of ethnomedicine, rooted in a particular cultural and historical setting.

 Activity 7.1

Go back to Chapter 1 and re-read the section on the anthropological concept of culture. Also have another look at the section on comparison and difference in Chapter 2. Then read the abridged excerpt below from Rhodes (1996).

Clifford Geertz suggests that cultural systems can best be understood in terms of their capacity to express the nature of the world and to shape that world. Thus, for example, religion 'formulates, by means of symbols, an image of a genuine order of the world.' This simultaneous shaping and expression produces a congruence between culture and experience that provides an 'aura of factuality' within which cultural systems 'make sense' and seem 'uniquely real' to their participants. The implication is that cultural systems achieve a feeling of realness, that is, in part or whole, a by-product of their symbolic forms.

In Western society biomedicine is generally believed to operate in a realm of 'facts'. This realm of bodily fact is often perceived to be quite separate from other cultural and social domains. Given this assumption that nature and the body exist in a directly apprehendable realm of fact, the problem for a cultural analysis of biomedicine is the delineation of the 'aura' in the 'aura of factuality' that it promotes. The issue is not simply the description of biomedicine but the discovery of strategies that will make visible its nature as a cultural system. It takes a 'jolt' to see the 'contingent nature' of biomedical description.

Several recent explorations of biomedicine undertake specific and deliberate strategies to provide this jolt by making visible the culture of biomedicine. One strategy is historical contextualization; biomedicine is shown as the historically embedded product of particular cultural and social assumptions. Another strategy is to uncover, through analysis of metaphor and other forms of speech, ways in which social meaning is embedded in biomedical categories.

Attending to the life worlds of clinicians is a third strategy; the daily practice of clinicians is revealing of biomedicine's theoretical and pragmatic foundations. All of these forms of analysis aim to recover from the domain of the 'natural' and the 'given' those aspects of biomedicine that are cultural and constructed.

Most historical discussions of biomedicine emphasize its origin in an elaboration of the Cartesian dichotomy between mind and body. The body, as part of the natural world, becomes knowable as a bounded material entity; diseases similarly are physical entities occurring in specific locations within the body. This medicine also radically separates body from non body; the body is thought to be knowable and treatable in isolation.

The particularity of this way of knowing the body can be seen in biomedical texts and practices that provide a mechanistic and desocialised imagery of bodily processes. For example, in a section of her book *The Woman in the Body* (1987) Martin examines the images of women's bodies found in medical textbooks and suggests that several metaphors of the body permeate their seemingly 'scientific' (that is, in this context, neutral or value-free) descriptions of physical processes. Thus, the processes of menstruation and menopause are described in terms of production and control. The female reproductive system is geared to 'production' and is organized as a hierarchical system of communication among hormones, cells, and the brain. This imagery corresponds to that of our economic system. In menopause, 'what is being described is the breakdown of a system of authority . . . at every point in this system, functions "fail" and "falter." Follicles "fail to muster strength" to reach ovulation. As functions fail, so do the members of the system decline'. In these images, the 'natural' functioning of the body is described in a way that fits a wider social view of women as defined by their reproductive function.

A revealing account of the historical embeddedness of biomedical knowledge is provided by Michel Foucault. Foucault argues that modern medicine had its birth in the period around 1800 when medicine became clinically based and concerned with both the inside of the body and the control of the health of populations. Foucault describes the period around 1800 as one in which medicine shifted not from a less to a more accurate understanding of the body but from one kind of knowledge to another. Before 1800 Europe had a 'medicine of species' that depended on classification; diseases were organized into families and species and related more to one another than to the body of the patient. Medicine after 1800 was dominated by what Foucault calls 'the gaze,' a new way of seeing that looked into the body and focused on what was individual and abnormal.

Suddenly doctors were able to see and to describe what for centuries had been beneath the level of the visible. It was not so much that doctors suddenly opened their eyes; rather the old codes of knowledge had determined what was seen. A new way of seeing produced a new kind of knowledge: 'clinical experience sees a new space opening up before it; the tangible space of the body . . . the medicine of organs, sites, causes, a clinic wholly ordered in accordance with pathological anatomy' (Foucault 1975: 122).

For Foucault the historical context, and particularly its shaping of what is possible, of what can be seen, determines what at any time is considered to be true. Practitioners of the early nineteenth century did not suddenly become better observers and therefore better able to discover the truth about the body; rather, there was a fundamental change in what constituted observation. This change brought about profound changes in medicine, and these in turn shape the body we perceive. In this argument, the issue of shaping goes deeper than what is said. Foucault is interested in what can be said and in the mutual shaping of perception and possibility that gives rise to a particular medicine at a particular historical moment.

The assumption behind Geertz's definition of a cultural system is that 'culture can be explained primarily in terms of itself'. However, these examples suggest that the culture of biomedicine does not lend itself to explanation in terms of itself. One problem is the relationship between constructed and natural fact. Hahn points out that social science observers in biomedical settings have often paid insufficient attention to its materiality. Biomedical practice depends on the assumption of an objectified nature subject to scientifically formulated 'reality testing,' and although reality testing is fundamental to all healing traditions, we find our particular brand especially compelling. Thus, from the perspective of patients, practitioners, social scientists, and laypeople in our society and despite much evidence of limitations or confusion, nature as it is understood by biomedicine demands to be taken seriously (that is, not questioned) in studies of biomedicine. This paradox, usually not in evidence in studies of other medical systems, means that the categories of the culture under study are also the categories used to study it.

A second difficulty arises not so much in connection with factuality as with its aura. The closed circle of belief and expression suggested by the notion of cultural system appears flawed, even fragile, in several of these accounts. This may result in part from the way illness itself threatens the cultural order with chaos and loss of meaning and thus 'calls into question particular socio-cultural resolutions' of the dilemmas of human existence.

In addition, however, biomedicine participates in a cultural separation of mind and body, nature and culture, in ways that may produce a sense of dissonance expressed in increasing criticism and doubt. Martin, for example, found that women she interviewed expressed diverse images of their bodily processes, contradicting and resisting biomedical formulations. Thus, as Jean Comaroff puts it, 'there has been an awareness that "factual" knowledge might imply social values, that medicine has bequeathed us powerful metaphors along with its "natural" truths and that these might . . . reinforce the deep-seated paradoxes raised by illness.'

In what ways can we become aware of the cultural nature of biomedicine? Think about what we said in Chapter 1 about the concept of culture, and in Chapter 2 about comparison and difference. If necessary, re-read the excerpt again with this question in mind. Can you think of any other ways?

↻ Feedback

As we discussed in Chapter 1, anthropology studies 'the other', because focusing on different ways of doing things and different assumptions about the nature of things (reality) makes us aware that what we take for granted and assume to be common sense or universal is often culturally and historically situated. We can get an idea of the situatedness of biomedicine by studying other medical systems, seeing their 'cultural' character, and then seeking similar traits in biomedicine. This is easier said than done however, as biomedicine (like certain other Western 'cultural systems' – law, parliamentary democracy, human rights) has an obviousness for insiders that it is difficult to question. What is 'cultural' about having pneumonia and wanting antibiotic treatment that works? Surely these are hard objective facts?

In order to see the situatedness of biomedicine, Rhodes argues, we need a 'jolt' – something that makes us see, suddenly, that categories, assumptions, ways of seeing that we have taken for granted, are not so obvious after all. Recall here the discussion in Chapter 2 about the role of difference and comparison in anthropology.

One way of doing this is through historical contextualization. Rhodes briefly discusses the work of Foucault on how the way in which medicine viewed the body changed after 1800. The study of history also shows that the separation of the physical body from the mental and the social – a separation that has long been taken for granted in biomedicine and in Western thought more generally – was also a historical event, with its roots in the philosophy of the French philosopher René Descartes (1596–1650). A similar experience can be had by reading any history of medicine. For example, in *The Rise and Fall of Modern Medicine* (1999), James le Fanu shows how, up until relatively recently, it was quite normal for doctors to try out new medicines on their patients, whereas today it is unthinkable not to have to go through numerous phases of randomized controlled trials and obtain approval from countless regulatory bodies before any new pharmaceutical can be put on the market.

A second way of situating biomedicine is by studying the forms of speech used in biomedicine in order to uncover the ways is which social meanings are embedded in biomedical categories. Rhodes illustrates this by referring, among other things, to Emily

Martin's study of the images of women in medical textbooks, showing how what are ostensibly neutral, objective, scientific descriptions are in fact constructed using social metaphors that carry strong economic connotations of 'functionlessness'.

A third way of situating biomedicine is to study closely the actual daily practice of doctors (and, we might add, other medical practitioners).

Biomedicine's cultural nature also emerges from a consideration of the pluralism of different medical traditions existing side-by-side, or mixed together syncretically, and from the plurality within biomedicine itself – think of the difference between primary care practitioners in a rural health centre, brain surgeons in an academic teaching hospital, military health planners, nursing home nurses. It also becomes clear from reflection on national variations in biomedicine. For example, differences in the incidence of unnecessary surgical procedures between Europe and the United States, or Dutch bewilderment at the highly emotional Anglo-Saxon resistance to voluntary euthanasia. The cultural nature of biomedicine also emerges when we study changes in biomedicine (or perhaps the emergence of different biomedicines) resulting from indigenization, globalization and syncretism.

Bracketing biomedicine

The form of the relationship between anthropology and medicine that is probably most familiar to health professionals is that of the (subordinate) anthropologist employed by health professionals or medical researchers to work in a medical or public health setting on problems defined largely (and usually exclusively) by the former. For example, much of the social science research carried out in programmes and interventions relating to infectious diseases (for example, research aimed at revealing barriers to condom use, attitudes and beliefs relating to HIV/AIDS, risk behaviours and so forth) falls into this category. Here anthropology is largely uncritical of biomedicine, either because the anthropologist shares biomedical assumptions and priorities, or because he or she is constrained by the biomedical setting from investigating what biomedicine deems obvious. In all these settings, the anthropologist 'brackets' biomedicine by situating it outside the area covered by anthropological scrutiny.

Activity 7.2

Now re-read the section on the distinction between illness and disease in Chapter 4. Then read the following excerpt from Rhodes (1996):

One solution to the problem posed by medicine's grounding in 'fact' is to segregate biomedical and social science ways of knowing. Most of clinically applied anthropology, and much research in medical anthropology as a whole, is based on a bracketing of biomedical expertise as referring to areas of knowledge not within the purview of the anthropologist.

This bracketing is the basis for the well-known distinction between disease and illness. Thus illness includes the experiences and beliefs of individuals; disease is what biomedicine discovers 'in' the person regardless of his or her (personal or cultural) awareness. The disease-illness distinction has provided the basis for much work in medical anthropology on the explanatory models and semantic illness networks of patients and, to some extent, of practitioners. These studies set aside the disease half of the distinction and concentrate on understanding the illness experiences and behaviour of individuals and cultural groups. By 'setting aside,' I do not mean that disease itself is not considered problematic for those who experience it but that the definition of disease – its status as a real, natural phenomenon is considered nonproblematic. This has allowed medical anthropologists to study culture (beliefs, issues of meaning, experience of illness) in medical settings without dealing with questions of the cultural construction of medicine itself. It also allows for the defining of research problems (for example, the study of groups of patients suffering from a particular disease or the study of the relationship between cultural and physical aspects of causation in a particular disorder) in ways that are relevant to the social context supporting the research.

One consequence is that medical anthropologists have been able to do research and teaching in medical settings, finding ways to incorporate anthropology into practice while respecting the orientation and commitments of clinicians. For the anthropologist who is bicultural in anthropology and medicine, the ideal is a translation of perspectives, enabling clinicians to make use of anthropological insights. Often these insights have to do with negotiation among perspectives (as in, for example, Kleinman's use of explanatory models); at other times they have to do with patient advocacy or with the clarification of ways that the biomedical perspective influences the cultural interpretations of patients.

On the other hand, the disease-illness distinction is a variant of the mind-body and culture-nature dichotomies. By using it to separate natural facts from cultural constructions, medical anthropology runs the risk of taking on characteristics of biomedicine itself. Instead of offering a perspective that comes from a position of stranger, the anthropologist may be a kissing cousin in disguise. For example, the emphasis on case studies reproduces in anthropology the individual-centred and 'objective' approach of the medical case study. Similarly, the use of scientific language to describe disease reproduces the position 'from the outside looking over or into a space' that is fundamental to the medical gaze. The anthropologist is also influenced by the premise of biomedicine that 'it is *the* medicine, real medicine; only other ethnomedicines are specially denominated, "osteopathic medicine," "Chinese medicine" '. In both biomedical settings and the study of other kinds of medicine, it is hard to avoid the assumption that what needs to be explained are the 'alternatives,' the 'other' perspectives, the 'misunderstandings' or 'misuses' of biomedicine rather than biomedicine itself.

An interesting recent development is that as biomedicine expands its definitions of physical disorder, incorporating problems with recognizably large social components (for example, alcoholism and posttraumatic stress disorder), the position of the anthropologist becomes problematic. These conditions, with their roots in problematic social environments, seem to be ripe for anthropological analysis and understanding. However, attempts to bring social and cultural considerations to bear on biological phenomena tend to participate, often unwittingly, in a process of naturalization that turns them into things comparable to diseases.

The bringing of chronic or behavioural conditions into the domain of biomedical treatment (the very thing that brings them to the attention of the biomedically based medical anthropologist) tends to result in their naturalization and 'reinterpretation as events requiring medical intervention.' Thus, the more they are translated into the reified, concrete terminology of 'disorders,' the less room there is for the anthropologist's perspective on the cultural shaping of both the symptoms and their interpretation. As Alan Young has shown for posttraumatic stress disorder, the production of 'knowledge' about such disorders is itself a cultural process (Young 1988).

1 How does the idea of bracketing biomedicine in anthropological research on sickness relate to the distinction between illness and disease? How does this enhance the collaboration between anthropology and medicine?
2 Re-read the sections in Chapter 4 in which the phenomenon of medicalization is discussed. What are the consequences of medicalization for the anthropological bracketing of biomedicine?

Feedback

1 Dividing sickness into illness and disease enables disease to be bracketed as outside the domain of anthropology and allows the anthropologist to focus on one aspect of sickness while avoiding a critical evaluation of the what biomedicine defines as the 'real' problem. This 'division of labour' facilitates collaboration because the anthropologist can concentrate on the 'sociocultural' aspects of sickness for which doctors have no time but about which they would often like to know more (because they are seen as barriers to adherence, for example) without having to be critical of biomedicine or threaten the hegemony of the doctor in defining what is 'real'.

2 Through medicalization problematic aspects of the social domain are increasingly redefined as medical problems – even as disease – thus 'naturalizing' them. This brings both the study of their putative causes and the formulation of solutions into the purview of biomedicine, thus reducing the scope for an anthropological perspective on how the problem in question is socially and culturally determined.

Critique of biomedicine

The anthropologist can also take a distanced, critical view of biomedicine. A central concept here is *mystification*. Karl Marx famously referred to religion as the 'opium of the people'. By this he meant that religion, like opium, befuddled the mind so that once under its influence people are unable to see things for what they really are, and they then mistake their distorted view of reality for reality itself (compare this with the idea of 'cultural system' discussed above). Mystification not only hides the nature of reality but also serves to maintain the status quo and to protect those in power from criticism. For example religion, by representing political power in terms of sacredness (the divine right of kings, for instance) and defining power as supernaturally conferred, thus legitimates the exercise of power by certain individuals or groups over the rest of the population. As a result, we need to 'look *through* cultural conceptualisations as well as *at* them. Beneath symbolic systems, beneath ideas about sacredness and purity and religious duty, we need to see the realities of power: who has it, who uses it, in what ways, to what ends' (Keesing and Strathern 1998).

Basically, in this approach, biomedicine is seen as mystifying social, economic and political problems by making them appear individual, biological, natural. It hides (or ignores) the social causes of sickness (thus legitimizing the unequal distribution of sickness and resources and suppressing possible protest – think back to Paul Farmer's discussion of HIV/AIDS in Haiti). Critical medical anthropology (or political-economic medical anthropology, as it is also known) sees its task as 'looking through' biomedical mystifications, in order to show them for what they really are, and to reveal the interests that they serve.

In line with the concept of mystification, the discourse of critical medical anthropology is often shot through with a Marxist idiom of struggle and liberation. Thus Nancy Scheper-Hughes compares the relationship between (applied) medical anthropology and medicine to the earlier relationship between anthropology and colonialism, and suggests that in certain settings doctors are more like jailers to their patients than healers, while Soheir Morsy writes of critical anthropology 'liberating' us from medicalization (Scheper-Hughes 1990; Morsy 1996).

✎ Activity 7.3

Now read the third abridged excerpt from the article by Rhodes (1996). Here she discusses critical medical anthropology.

📖 Much work in anthropology has explored the positive aspects of cultural systems in providing and sustaining meaning in human social life. But there is another perspective from which the congruence between the shaping and expressive aspects of culture can be seen as perverse. Religion, for example, appears in this view as an 'opiate,' preventing people from recognizing the truth of their situation. Medicine, in its powerful mediation of human physical and emotional frailty, can similarly be understood in terms of its relationship to a larger social (political and economic) system in which it serves to conceal sources of injustice and suffering. From this point of view, medicine cannot be described apart from the relations of power that constitute its social context. As Howard Waitzkin puts it: 'Major problems in medicine are also problems of society; the health system is so intimately tied to the broader society that attempts to study one without the other are misleading. Difficulties in health and medical care emerge from social contradictions and rarely can be separated from those contradictions' (Waitzkin 1983).

There are two aspects to this relationship. One is that health problems themselves may be socially caused, creating what Waitzkin calls the 'second sickness'. The other, related, aspect is that medicine may function to conceal the social origins of sickness and to suppress the possibility of protest.

When biomedicine is seen in this light, clinical knowledge itself becomes problematic; its connections to the larger system mean that it 'cannot be either evaluated or transformed in any simple, decontextualized manner'. Nor can it be seen merely as a 'web of significance,' approachable through understanding; it must also (or perhaps, instead) be considered as a 'web of mystification'.

Critical analyses of biomedicine are attempts at demystification. One strategy aims to uncover the incidence and causes of the 'second sickness' by exploring ways in which medical care fails to reach, recognize, or correct socially created problems. Many analyses stress the relationship between capitalist production (and the profit motive inherent in it) and the failure to protect workers and others from its effects. Others focus on the maldistribution of medical care and the effects on the health of populations created by the dominance of complex technology.

A second strategy aims to uncover how biomedicine mystifies sickness through its participation in the nature-culture dichotomy.

Medicine, because of its bias toward the uncovering of natural facts, represents the body in ways that are powerfully suggestive of a natural reality separate from the social. The effect, if not the intention, is to make the social invisible and to place sickness, as a natural process or entity, inside the individual.

Martin's point in her argument about menopause is that the 'shriveling' of the ovaries is a metaphor that rests on and reinforces the social representation of the 'shriveling' of production in the older woman. Because medicine has clothed the social representation in scientific language, it is difficult to discover its origins. By placing the body and bodily experience in the realm of nature, biomedicine conceals both the social causes of sickness and the social embeddedness of the experience of sickness. Thus, for example, the diagnostic category of premenstrual syndrome (PMS) creates a 'disorder' that may serve to obscure the social relations that are the context of women's suffering. Similarly, the processes of childbirth and dying may be isolated from their social contexts and treated in largely technical terms that prevent those involved from taking care of themselves and each other.

Recent cross-cultural and historical studies suggest that these tendencies toward reification and mystification are widely associated with biomedical practice. Lock's work on school refusal and on menopause in Japan shows that Japanese biomedicine similarly describes social problems as 'syndromes' to be treated (Lock 1986). In northeast Brazil, medical treatment, especially in the form of tranquilizers, serves to conceal the economic and social origin of starvation (Scheper-Hughes 1992). Other areas of medicine have also been seen as fostering dependence in order to conceal and support class and gender interests. The notion of the body as a mechanism that could be repaired corresponded in important ways to factory production. Similarly, nineteenth-century medical theories about the fragility and emotionality of women served to bolster male dominance and the creation of the home as a domain separate from the workplace.

These analyses regard biomedicine's aura of factuality as precisely its source of power. Medicine can describe events in a value-neutral language that makes them appear to be part of the natural world and thus neutralizes what are, in reality, social problems. In the nineteenth century, villagers whose ability to support aging relatives had been undermined by social change were convinced that asylum care was provided by 'experts' (doctors) and thus superior to their own; women who rebelled against restrictive conditions could be persuaded that bed rest was the only remedy for their restless female organs. Similarly, today, Brazilian peasants believe tranquilizers to be 'medicine' for starvation, and women angry over the unfair distribution of domestic work regard their anger as a 'symptom' of PMS.

For some writers this analysis of the embeddedness of biomedical categories in social life (and their tendency to perpetuate sickness-causing aspects of social life) is not enough. Additionally, it is important to recognize the ways in which biomedicine also gives rise to resistance. Martin attempts to make visible, through the analysis of women's speech, the way ordinary women resist the biomedical description of women's bodily life. For example, women may refuse to go to the hospital for childbirth, or they create original metaphors to describe bodily processes. Those who emphasize the misuse of medicine are more prescriptive. If the problem is the creation of sickness under capitalism and the maldistribution and misappropriation of biomedicine, then the solution does not lie so much with changes in biomedicine itself or with pockets of resistance among patients or practitioners as in larger-scale changes in the system. Criticism of biomedicine – regardless of whether the stress is on discovering resistance or creating a new system – often seems to involve a paradox. On the one hand biomedicine as part of society is seen as failing to serve the real best interests of that society. On the other hand, the techniques of biomedicine (its science) are seen as one means for discovering these real best interests.

In some instances, biomedical categories themselves are employed to critique the use of biomedicine. For instance, Nancy Scheper-Hughes uses biomedical definitions of starvation to challenge the misuse of biomedicine to conceal it. This sidesteps the question, raised by those who consistently question biomedical categories (for example, Foucault), as to whether the science of biomedicine itself does not contain intrinsic assumptions about society and about the nature of reality that are, at best, disempowering and, at worst, harmful to body and society (as in, for example, Ivan Illich's critique of medicine's iatrogenic effects (Illich 1976)).

Now answer the following questions:

1 How does critical anthropology claim to demystify biomedicine?
2 What does Rhodes see as the paradox involved in the criticism of biomedicine?
    How do you think this can be avoided?

↻ Feedback

1 First, by studying the incidence of socially created sickness, and the unequal distribution of sickness and medical care. Second, by uncovering the social nature of medical categories and descriptions – for example, by revealing how the creation of the disorder of premenstrual syndrome serves to obscure the social relations that are the real cause of women's suffering, or the way in which the prescription of tranquillizers to poor women conceals the social origin of poverty and starvation. Third, by uncovering the historical roots of biomedicine's underlying assumptions.

2 On the one hand biomedicine fails to address the real problems in society (poverty, inequality, exploitation) while concealing them behind medical categories, but at the

same time biomedicine and its categories are a means of identifying these problems (poverty and inequality are expressed as *disease* – as biomedically defined). To avoid this paradox would require adopting a critical stance toward critical medical anthropology itself, situating it as we situate biomedicine.

Summary

In this chapter we have presented the argument that biomedicine is a cultural system – culturally determined rather than neutral and objective – and should therefore be viewed critically as one among many ethnomedicines. This leads to the question whether anthropology and biomedicine can collaborate productively and, if so, in what way. One of the options we have discussed is bracketing biomedicine (thus bypassing the question of biomedicine's claims to legitimacy). This is made easier by the obvious advantages of biomedicine over other medical traditions. This approach need not be uncritical of biomedicine, as we have seen in the case of Paul Farmer. Farmer accepts biomedical disease categories (such as HIV/ AIDS) as objective and given (as do many of the more critical anthropologists) and attempts – as physician and anthropologist – to alleviate suffering. But at the same time he is critical of biomedicine and its neglect of the wider issues of structural violence. So although anthropology must maintain a critical stance, there is scope for collaboration.

References

Foucault M (1975) *The Birth of the Clinic: An Archeology of Medical Perception*. New York: Vintage.

Illich I (1976) *Medical Nemisis. The Expropriation of Health*. London: Calder & Boyars.

Keesing RM and Strathern AJ (1998) *Cultural Anthropology. A Contemporary Perspective*. New York: Holt, Rinehart & Winston.

Kleinman A (1995) *Writing at the Margin. Discourse Between Anthropology and Medicine*. Berkeley: University of California Press.

Le Fanu J (1999) *The Rise and Fall of Modern Medicine*. London: Abacus.

Lock M (1986) Plea for acceptance: school refusal syndrome in Japan. *Social Science and Medicine* 23: 99–112.

Martin E (1987) *The Woman in the Body: A Cultural Analysis of Reproduction*. Boston: Beacon Press.

Morsy S (1996) Political economy in medical anthropology, in Sargent C and Johnson T (eds) *Medical Anthropology. Contemporary Theory and Method*. Westport: Praeger.

Rhodes L (1996) Studying biomedicine as a cultural system, in Sargent C and Johnson T (eds) *Medical Anthropology. Contemporary Theory and Method*. Westport: Praeger.

Scheper-Hughes N (1990) Three propositions for a critically applied medical anthropology. *Social Science and Medicine* 30: 189–97.

Scheper-Hughes N (1992) *Death Without Weeping: The Violence of Everyday Life in Brazil*. Berkeley: University of California Press.

Waitzkin H (1983) *The Second Sickness: Contradictions of Capitalist Health Care*. New York: Free Press.

Young A (1988) A description of how ideology shapes knowledge of a mental disorder, in Lindenbaum S and Lock M (eds) *Analysis in Medical Anthropology*. Dordrecht: Kluwer.

8 Substances of power

Overview

The aim of this chapter is to examine 'medicines' as powerful, transformational substances. In this sense, Western pharmaceuticals are not only chemical substances but also social and cultural objects with diverse and often contradictory meanings and uses. We start with a discussion of the anthropological approach to medicines in this sense. Then, referring back to earlier discussions of medical systems in Chapter 4 and the criticism of patient agency in Chapter 6, we explore the search for health from the practical point of view of the users, with an example from south India. Finally, we examine the popularity of pharmaceuticals by showing how they are given different (non-biomedical), social meanings.

Learning objectives

By the end of this chapter you should be able to

- **appreciate the variety of meanings that can be given to medicines**
- **consider the implications of medicines' mobility and varying meanings for public health**

Key terms

Medicine Substances (or objects) that, based on their inherent potency, are employed to engender transformations, such as the bodily change from ill-health to health.

Pharmaceutical Medicine that is based on biomedical knowledge and industrially produced.

The anthropological study of medicines

Until the end of the 1980s, anthropologists studied medicines mainly by examining non-Western people's 'traditional' remedies, often with the aim of evaluating their biomedical efficacy. Some anthropologists combined their concern with social life with attention to botany, such as Victor Turner's seminal work on the symbolism of southern African plant medicines (1967), which employed botanical knowledge to produce knowledge of ritual, society and culture. Such rigorous studies of herbal medicines and their meanings are extremely valuable. Here, we propose a slightly different angle, studying medicines themselves, including what used to be distinguished as traditional and Western medicines, as social and cultural phenomena (Whyte *et al.* 2002).

All medical traditions make use of things, medicines, to engender transformations to more desirable states: from illness to health, towards outcomes such as growth, fertility or the birth of a child, or from one life stage to another, such as when medicines are used in initiation, betrothal or burial. Medicines can even engender transformations outside the human body, such as the growth and health of live-stock or crops, or the fruitfulness of the land or the weather. The crucial point that links all these 'medicines' is that the capacity to elicit transformation lies within the substance or thing. As such, in most general terms, medicines are powerful substances.

As powerful substances, medicines attract attention and are given meanings. Their outer form and their hidden capacities provoke people's imagination. Such creativity is situated in specific social contexts and thus every medicine is given particular, often varying and changing, meanings in any given context, producing a multiplicity of ideas and of practices. In turn, diverse ideas and meanings influence what the powerful substances do. One way in which meaning influences the work of medicines is widely known as the placebo effect (Moerman 2000): medicines' capacity to transform people's health state and experience is in part independent of their scientifically proven pharmacological efficacy. For example, a patient who unknowingly receives an injection with saline solution, might nevertheless feel better or improve, because he attributes power to the injection or the administering doctor. This 'meaning effect', which is part of any medicine use, underlines that there is more to medicines than their pharmacological properties, that their work is co-produced by a context of meanings and social relations.

Medicines, being things, can be detached from the human relations that produced them; they can move faster between social and cultural contexts than the traditions of medical knowledge from which they are derived. If recognized as medicine, they will still be regarded as potent, but ideas about what they are good for and how they work might change. Being things, medicines move, carry along or leave behind meanings and relations, and take on new ones in each new context. As such, they provide nodes around which we can explore transformations of medicine, health, the body and society.

The broad meanings of the term 'medicine' as powerful substance can be illustrated with the East African Kiswahili term *dawa*. *Dawa* can refer to almost any substance or object with the capacity to change things: herbs and pharmaceuticals, injections and sorcery objects, engine fuel and battery acid, insecticides and industrial fertilizer, marihuana and food preservatives. The power of *dawa* derives from a source that cannot be entirely controlled, from outside the common, visible world, such as the world of spirits or ancestors, a neighbouring tribe, a factory or Europe. The fact that medicines contain the capacity to change persons and bodies, even to give life, and that this power cannot entirely be harnessed, means that medicines are ambivalent: they can do good and evil; save lives and kill. *Dawa* groups biomedical pharmaceuticals together with a range of substances; their meanings inform each other, creating a social and cultural field which is more complex than one, from a biomedical perspective, would associate with the category 'medicine'.

This categorization is important for medical anthropologists working in public health, because people's associations – say between pharmaceuticals and poisons, or insecticides and sorcery-substances – which transcend the boundaries of public health thinking may well explain some of people's responses to public health interventions. Where a public health worker sees the positive side of medical interventions such as vaccination campaigns, a person reasoning in the broader frame of *dawa* asks: what is the other side of it, the danger, the potential evil? Public health workers tend to reason in terms of problems (an epidemic) and solutions (a treatment campaign); they react with surprise if the beneficiaries of their interventions, considering the equivocal, undetermined potency of *dawa*, show moderate enthusiasm for their solutions.

To acknowledge the breadth of emic understandings of medicines is useful to make sense of and engage with local responses to health interventions. Beyond this applied scope, the analytical focus on 'powerful, transformative and ambiguous, substances' also helps the understanding of public health and health systems. The pharmaceuticals that biomedical interventions often rest on are more than what a laboratory has put into them. They are small nodes around which meanings coagulate, and which, along their movements, create ever new connections between people, places and knowledges. By examining these nodes, medical anthropologists can study the larger networks or systems.

Meanings of medicines

Anthropologists in public health often have to explain what people do in response to an illness, and why they do not do what would be most beneficial from a public health perspective (and how they can be induced to do so). There are certain obvious factors, such as affordability or availability of health services, but even hard-and-fast economic facts can be variously interpreted. For example, many people in Kenya find a 20 KSh (20 British pence) user fee at a health facility too expensive, but would sell a cow to pay a diviner 5000 KSh to identify an illness. There has been a tendency to present such issues as a matter of choice between therapy systems: patients, as an individual agents, choose the system they favour based on their own explanations of illness (which they, in turn, choose from those offered by medical pluralism).

There are several arguments against such reasoning, which were presented in some detail above: (a) the notion of medical system suggests internal coherence and clear boundaries towards other systems, which from the patient's point of view might not be so (see Chapter 4); (b) the model of 'choice' assumes rational decision making, which does not adequately reflect what happens in practice and how knowledge translates into action (Chapter 6); (c) the notion of individual choice might be inappropriate where people decide together and where the notion of autonomous action does not fit (let alone contexts where conditions of life leave precious little choice at all) (Chapter 6). This misrepresentation of health seeking and its determinants results from looking at things from a biomedical perspective, in which medical systems are viewed as separate, and in which patients represent individual sick bodies and individual healing agents.

These shortcomings can be remedied by looking at the 'things', the medicines, and exploring the search for health from the practical point of view of the users. What do the medicines look like, how do they taste, and how do their qualities fit into wider understandings of body and health? In this way, the supposed boundaries of systems are suspended, and meanings, interpretations, contexts can be explored.

Activity 8.1

Read the abridged extract from Nichter (1996) below. As you read it, consider:

1 What meanings are attributed to pharmaceuticals and what implications do these have for their use?
2 Similar examples of non-biomedical meanings of pharmaceuticals that shape their use.
3 What the anthropology of medicines contributes to public health?

Popular perceptions of medicine: a south Indian case study

Introduction

In this chapter, I explore popular perceptions of medicine in South Kanara District, Karnataka State, India. My analysis will question the widespread portrayal of the rural villager as thinking within a coherent Ayurvedic classic Indian medicine cognitive framework, and reveal the eclectic practice of medicine in India and the mix of medicines produced and available to the public. I argue that the type of therapy system to which a practitioner is affiliated often matters less to patients than the form and qualities of medicines he dispenses. I document how medicine appropriateness is evaluated both in terms of illness and patient characteristics. The afflicted's relative strength, age, previous experience with medicine, and special disposition all influence perceptions of medicine suitability.

Ayurveda and popular health culture

The background of medicinal practice in South Kanara is the Ayurveda, but not in the sense of a coherent 'system': to most villagers it is only known partially, practitioners mix it with other medicines, e.g. biomedicine, and many Ayurvedic medicines have been industrialised and adapted to biomedical terminology in an attempt to 'scientize' Ayurveda while simultaneously emphasizing Ayurveda's long, glorious, and sacred tradition. Popular health culture in India is a bricolage, an assemblage of eclectic conceptual and material resources.

Masala medicine in the health bazaar

When searching for treatment of acute complaints, rural South Indian villagers are attentive to the cost of therapy, practitioner availability, and practitioner reputation irrespective of the type of therapy system or training course to which they are formally affiliated. A trial and error approach to the seeking of treatment is common. Given this environment, many practitioners feel compelled to adapt their practice of medicine to client demands. Client demands often take the form of illness and age specific preferences for forms of medicine associated with ideas about medicine habituation, compatibility, and power.

Habituation

An appreciation of habituation *abhyasa* is important for an understanding of medicine-taking behaviour. It is common to hear villagers describing that a medicine has not been effective because they have no *abhyasa* for that kind of medicine. According to local reasoning, in order for the body to 'take to' a new food or type of medicine, it must first adjust to its properties. In the case of medicine, a young child regularly receives herbal medicines to promote health and prevent a number of culturally defined illnesses.

Cosmopolitan biomedical medicine is generally not administered to a child until an illness crisis occurs. Cosmopolitan medicines are thought to be too powerful for a young child's body to be able to accommodate. Moreover, it is thought that they interfere with a child's capacity to 'take to' the herbal medicines used in the home for preventive as well as curative purposes. Children are gradually introduced to cosmopolitan medicine during an illness crisis wherein it is deemed prudent to manage serious symptoms by English medicine. Over time, it is thought that frequent consumption of English medicine causes the user to lose their habituation to herbal medicine and gain habituation to cosmopolitan medicine.

Many villagers think that English medicine offers a quick cure, but harms one's body and undermines one's health over time. This concern is expressed in different ways. Some people speak of English medicine as heating while others say its continued use leads to bloodlessness and weakness. There is a second meaning conveyed by the comment that the use of English medicine leads to weakness. Developing an *abhyasa* to English medicine, entails entering into a dependency relationship.

An increasing number of villagers have come to question the long-term utility of English medicines, especially fixes which appear to require continual or repeated use. In some cases this is because only symptomatic treatment is being offered to them, not a cure.

People may return to using herbal medicine for several reasons. Patients who have an ailment which cosmopolitan medicine has failed to cure may consume blood purifiers, purgatives and diuretics to cleanse the body and prepare themselves for herbal treatment. Other people seek herbal medicine which will enhance their body's ability to respond to English medicine after they have noticed a decline in the response of the allopathic medicines they have been taking for a chronic illness. Some people think it is harmful to take English medicine every day and so suspend treatment temporarily until symptoms flare up, while others approach Ayurvedic practitioners for medicines to improve the body's ability to 'digest' English medicines.

Meta-medical reasons also underlie the use of Ayurvedic medicines. Some people seek realignment with Ayurvedic medicine as a means of an identity reconstruction which entails the embodiment of 'Hindu' values. Among this group are the elderly preparing for a good death, as well as those in Hindu revivalist groups who champion Ayurveda for political as well as personal purposes. The taking of Ayurvedic medicines constitutes a means of affirming a moral identity. Consumption of such medicine provides a satisfying, empowering remedy for the pressures of modernization as well as an evocative, sensuous experience analogous to the eating of culturally marked foods which trigger a cascade of memories and associations.

Power

Comments about a medicine's power are common whenever therapy is discussed. Villagers consider medicine in relation to both its inherent power and their ability to accommodate to this power. Powerful medicine is desired by those whose body can stand the 'shock' associated with it. A medicine's shock effect is considered carefully when the afflicted is weak, when a chronic illness demands long-term treatment, or if a person is experiencing a heightened state of vulnerability such as during pregnancy or postpartum. Shock is also an important health concern influencing health care decisions involving infants and children rendered weak by multiple or long-term illness.

As a category, English medicines are spoken of as powerful yet dangerous. Power is regarded as unstable, vacillating, and requiring control. While English medicine is praised for its fast action, it is commonly spoken about as having 'uncontrolled' side effects. Ayurvedic medicine, on the other hand, is referred to as safe, and as establishing control and balance in the body 'causing no side effects.' English medicine is commonly referred to as heating and Ayurvedic medicine as neutral, although individual medicines within each system are recognized as having heating and cooling properties. The term 'heating' is multi vocal. Its meaning varies by context and indexes concepts related to strength, control, speed, and affect on the blood. Saying that English medicines are heating is, in one sense, a statement about the speed at which they act. It also indexes associations with uncontrolled activity and heightened danger. The term 'neutral,' when applied as a general descriptor of Ayurvedic medicine expresses balanced action and the concept of control. Stating that English medicine is heating also infers something about its perceived affect on the blood. The notion exists that heating the blood causes it to evaporate. The statement that English medicine is heating conveys a sense that one is at risk to general symptoms of malaise as well as symptoms such as burning skin, rashes, and burning urine. All of these symptoms are associated with excess heat in the body.

Some villagers frequent Ayurvedic practitioners or folk herbalists weeks or even months after taking English medicine for decoctions to cool the body and replenish blood which has been evaporated by excess heat in the body. Herbal medicine is taken as a complement to English medicine to restore the integrity of body process which powerful medicines have disrupted. The notion that powerful medicine disrupts body processes and causes weakness is one reason why English medicine is not favoured for the very young or old.

Perceptions of a medicine's properties and power influences the 'innovative' ways people use it. Medicines administered for one purpose are sometimes used for other purposes on the basis of assumptions about how they affect the body. For example, menses is thought to be a state of overheat in the body. When a woman suffers from amenorrhoea (lack of menses) a cosmopolitan practitioner or chemist shop attendant may offer her a hormone booster such as E. P. Forte to induce her period. The popular interpretation of the drug's action is that it causes the blood to heat up such that the wind inside the body pushes the blood outward.

Perceptions of the power of a medicine are related to both dose and medicine form. Tablets are generally perceived to be weaker doses of medication than injections or capsules. Capsules are stronger than pills but weaker than injections.

Perceptions of the power of medicine affect medicine self-regulation and supplementation. Some people try to enhance the power of recommended doses of medication. If one tablet does not yield satisfactory results, two or three tablets are taken simultaneously.

Physical characteristics of medicine

As mentioned earlier, the form in which a medicine is administered is highly significant to the villager. It is not uncommon to hear a patient request a liquid mixture, pills, or an injection during a consultation. Patients express interest in the colour and taste of medicines prescribed. Injections, as noted above, are considered powerful and heating. They are very popular, commonly requested and preferred by those who want quick symptomatic relief. For patients who fear that they may be too weak to withstand the shock of an injection, 'injection-powered pills' (capsules) are sometimes requested. For infants and those experiencing chronic debility and weakness, liquid mixtures are requested not only for ease in administration, but also because they are considered to be less powerful and 'shocking' to the body.

Preferences for medicine forms influence but do not determine health care seeking. In instances where dramatic curative action is required, health concerns may be temporarily suspended. Such cases do not necessarily have to be life threatening. For example, injections are not generally popular for toddlers. However, they are deemed especially effective for the treatment of infected wounds and rashes where pus is manifest and fear about swelling is expressed. The heating action of injections is thought to dry up infected, weeping rashes and wounds.

Among adults, a health concern associated with medicine taking is that medicine interferes with digestion, resulting in debility. Weakness experienced by a patient during an illness in which pills have been administered is often attributed to the pill's disruption of the patient's digestive process and not to the illness. If tablets cause thirst or a practitioner tells the patient to drink plenty of water with the tablet, the medication is suspected to be not only difficult to digest, but heating as well.

Private doctors are responsive to what they perceive to be patients' medicine preferences because they practice in a competitive health care arena. By being so, they reproduce impressions of what constitutes suitable medicines for particular illnesses and age groups. Pharmaceutical companies in turn are alert to the forms of medicines which doctors prescribe and purchase. Medicine supply and demand reinforce one another. Doctors attempt to meet patient preferences and patterns of medicine dispensing both respond to and foster popular demand.

Medicines are scrutinized in terms of colours since colours are thought to signify a medicine's inherent properties. For example, black medicines are thought to be powerful as well as good at reducing nausea, dizziness, or yellow bodily excretions. While black pills are considered appropriate for vomiting, fever, and fits, they are not appropriate for digestive disorders, weakness, or bloodlessness. This is one reason why black ferrous sulphate (iron) tablets are not popular among pregnant women and those experiencing weakness and anaemia. Both the form and colour of this iron supplement are not culturally appropriate for groups at risk to anaemia.

White medicines, particularly liquids, are generally attributed neutral or cooling qualities. They are thought to be more easily digested by the body than medicines of other colours and are trusted more when consumed for the first time. Because white pills are often interpreted as cooling, they are considered appropriate for fever, burning sensation, body pain, headache, and a loss of vitality – complaints all linked to an excess of heat in the body.

Red medicines have multiple connotations. For example, red pills are perceived to be heating and good for wet cough and cold. Liquid red medicines are thought to be blood producing, irrespective of whether they are classified as hot or cold. Yellow medicines are generally thought to be heating. As a topical medicine, however, yellow ointments are viewed as purification agents. An association is made between yellow and turmeric, a traditional blood and skin purifier used both in the home and for ritual purposes. Burnol, an ointment purchased over-the-counter, is used for a wide range of skin infections and cuts. Its popularity is in large part derived from its yellow colour, which villagers associate with turmeric. Here we have an instructive case where the attributes of a traditional medicine have been successfully applied to a commercial medicine with a similar physical characteristic.

Taste, like the form and colour of medicine, is also regarded as a sign of a medicine's inherent characteristics. Astringent and bitter tasting medicines are generally regarded as cooling for the body and are thought to have a positive promotive/ medicinal value. Herbs having a bitter/astringent taste are labeled bitter and are commonly used as folk medicines. Salty medicines, on the other hand, are viewed suspiciously by villagers and thought harmful for the bones (causing brittleness) if taken for any length of time. Pungent medicines are considered appropriate for cough (as they melt mucus) and as digestive aides, but they are considered inappropriate for skin diseases, urinary tract disorders, or rheumatic complaints.

Perceptions of the inherent lightness and heaviness of substances affect the way in which they are evaluated as curative resources. Light is a concept which connotes relative digestibility and low 'shock' impact on bodily processes. Those who are young, pregnant, weak, or convalescing are thought to require restorative medicines and supplements which are light and easy to digest. Healthy persons who wish to enhance their present state of health or improve their weight are attracted to medicines which are associated with heavy and strength producing substances. An important distinction is made between: 1) substances which are appropriate as resources promoting convalescence when one's digestive capacity is weak, and 2) medicines and foods promoting positive health when one's digestive capacity is strong. This distinction impacts on medicine-taking behaviour. Tonics and supplements are taken during illness and convalescence to protect digestive capacity as well as to provide nutrient resources. Products like glucose powder have become immensely popular in India as health supplements marketed as 'light' sources of energy which are easy to digest as opposed to sugar or jaggery which are considered to be heavy. This central concern in popular health culture – the digestibility of a product – is often highlighted in medicine advertisements.

Conclusion
I have focused on popular perceptions of medicine and illustrated how such perceptions underlie consumer demand and medicine taking practices. A greater appreciation of how medications are viewed by the lay population provides valuable insights into why illness, age, gender, and class-specific patterns of medicine-taking

behaviour exist. Such insights are clearly different from data generated by studies which focus on patterns of curative resort to 'therapy systems.' The latter place too much emphasis on 'system choice' and not enough on contingencies which lead people to use different types of medication, at different times, for different purposes. Moreover, studies of therapy systems have limited value in contexts where eclectic treatment is common and commercial forms of patent indigenous medicines are undistinguishable from allopathic medicine.

The ways in which popular ideas about medicine influence health care seeking, medicine compliance, and self-regulation are underappreciated by many in the international health field. In the field of medical anthropology, there has been a tendency to privilege explanatory models of illness when conducting ethnographic research. Explanatory models of medicines are just as important to consider as explanatory models of illness when studying health care behaviour. The two often influence one another in contexts where diagnosis by treatment is common and the type(s) of medicine prescribed and consumed mark illness severity as well as patient identity. At issue is not only what types of medicine are deemed appropriate for different illnesses, but which medicines are appropriate for different types of people.

It is prudent to consider what it is about specific types of medication, or combination of medications, which make them popular or unpopular for the treatment or prevention of a particular illness (or a range of illnesses). This is no simple task. It requires a broad based investigation of issues ranging from indigenous notions of ethnophysiology to colour symbolism, from cultural conceptualisations of power to health concerns related to medicines gleaned from the observation of other domains of life. Such study demands not only a consideration of medicines in and of themselves, but also of contingencies set up by medicine taking. As we have seen, advice given to patients by practitioners about medicines is often interpreted in relation to pre-existing conceptual frameworks which lend themselves to particular types of action.

What can contextualised studies of medication contribute to international health? Such studies are obviously relevant to social marketing approaches to popularising public health fixes. They are also important for health service research. If the types of medicine being distributed to high risk segments of the population are not being utilized, it is worth considering whether the characteristics of the medicines employed are deemed inappropriate, or whether it is the system of therapy which is unpopular for the task at hand. Studies of medicine-taking behaviour are also warranted if they help identify dangerous practices associated with popular misconceptions (and unrealistic expectations) about medications. This includes innovative ways drugs are used in keeping with perceptions about their inherent properties. Public health practitioners can also benefit from studies of medicine-taking behaviour which focus on perceptions of when medicines should and should not be taken. The timing of promotive and preventive health fixes impacts on their popularity beyond the issues of access, economics, and convenience.

While anthropologists can be an immense help in tailoring health intervention programs to local contexts, they must take care not to become party to simplistic or short sighted approaches to primary health care. This demands a fair degree of reflexivity and the viewing of problems and alternative solutions from a number of different vantage points. The focus of applied medical anthropological research on pharmaceutical practice must extend beyond the purview of compliance to a critical examination of social and economic factors driving both the distribution of medicines and information about these and other biotechnical fixes. In order to hold themselves accountable, anthropologists must look beyond solving immediate health service problems to the conditions which foster ill health and social resources available to alter these conditions.

Feedback

1 They are considered more powerful, but uncontrollable, potentially dangerous; tablets and injections could be 'shocking'; they heat the body; they reduce the blood; they are bad for digestion. Due to their strength, they are bad for weak people. This influences when and how medicines are used and by whom, and it explains polypharmacy, combining medicines with complementary meanings to attain a balance.

2 An example is the notion, among many people in western Kenya, that childhood sickness must 'come out' of the body as rashes or diarrhoea (see Chapter 10). Since pharmaceuticals and particularly injections are thought to 'push the illness back inside', they should never be used together with herbs that make it 'come out', as the contradiction would exacerbate the sickness.

3 To explore health seeking behaviour prior to health interventions; to prepare, advertise and time new health interventions. To identify misuse of medicine based on diverging meanings; to improve commercial advertising for medicines. To prevent simplistic approaches to public health; to foster respect for the diverse rationalities of different ways of using medicines.

The popularity of medicines

Despite the ambiguous meanings some people attribute to them, pharmaceuticals are universally popular. How do we explain their popularity? One, simple way is to point to their effectiveness compared to many herbal medicines; pharmaceuticals such as analgesics or antibiotics offer prompt relief from pain or cure of infections. Another dimension is their association with powerful other worlds, the wealth and dominance of industrial societies and the world of commodities. This explains why in many African countries, pharmaceuticals from distant, powerful and rich places such as the United States or Switzerland are considered more potent than those made in India, and the latter more powerful than those made in Africa. However, these factors cannot alone explain why pharmaceuticals bought in a shop are usually more popular than, say, operations performed at a government hospital, which are also linked to powerful outside worlds and knowledges. Why are *medicines* – pills one can buy – often more enthusiastically embraced than *medicine* – the social context and knowledge that makes biomedicine?

One of the reasons might be that a surgical operation is set in complex power relations, in which the patient is but a passive part, whereas pharmaceuticals give the patient the impression of being in control. Patients appear to be 'liberated' from the social relations within which healing and illness are commonly constituted, as they can decide when to buy which medicine and when to take it. Of course, this notion of choice in a world of commodities is an ideological representation of power relations that are hidden in the production and the exchange of medicines; if one considers who controls the making of drugs, their price, and whether a patient can afford to buy them or not, the imaginary freedom to choose becomes a rather narrow, prefigured catalogue (see Chapter 9). Yet, this imaginary of choice is powerful, precisely because of the illusion of freedom that it introduces into situations that are marked by a lack of it. As the manifold adverts for vitamins and power drinks in many Western countries suggest: if one cannot change one's employer's expectations and the lack of legislation to curb these, one can at least choose between an array of medicines in order to 'protect oneself', 'cope with life', 'avoid burning out' or 'regain strength'. Similarly, women in Eastern Africa use scarce resources on perfectly useless tonics for their babies, while many of the babies die due to communicable diseases; to buy the medicine is here an expression of motherly care, while none of the mothers could hope to change the economic conditions of child mortality itself.

By disentangling sickness from social relations, pharmaceuticals allow casting bodily suffering as a disease for which there is a medicine. An individual, autonomous health agent is produced, in tune with wider societal imaginations of 'consumers' and 'choice'. This supposed liberation contributes to the gradual deterioration of immediate and locally controlled social relations, and an increasing dependency of the individualised patients on the medical and economic systems that produce pharmaceuticals. Examples such as the increasing reliance of people in industrialised countries on the 'choice' of antidepressants or potency boosters point at the risk of such medicalisation and individualisation of social problems (see the seminal critique of medicalisation by Illich, 1976). On the other hand, commodified pharmaceuticals allow people in strained situations to disentangle themselves from the networks that they otherwise rely on in their struggle for health. For example, a mother in a village can buy a tablet for her child – if she has money – rather than engaging in a ritual governed by her mother-in-law or putting herself at the mercy of a powerful government doctor. Alongside a range of societal transformations that propagate values such as self-control, personal development, individual achievement, and autonomy, pharmaceuticals offer people control of their own body.

Despite their dangers, pharmaceuticals engender cultural productivity, and, irrespective of their intended or hidden effects, they provoke surprising social inventions. Being discrete things, one can employ pharmaceuticals on one's own, and, once they have been appropriated, pharmaceuticals can be put to different uses, in addition to treatment: as tokens of affection or relatedness, as gifts or as shared substances, or as signs of parental responsibility. In other words, one can do a lot with them, because they are (limited by their place in a capitalist commodity economy) mobile and malleable. This is the 'charm of medicines' that the anthropologists Sjaak Van der Geest and Susan R. Whyte were taken in by (see Van der Geest and Whyte 1989).

Summary

In this chapter we have seen how pharmaceuticals, far from being mere chemical substances, contain multiple and contradictory meanings and are integrated into different cultural and social contexts. We have seen how their 'thinginess' allows them to move and change contexts as well as their own meanings, and to constitute new connections. Thus, the stage is set for a complex interplay of people and things, substances, places and ideas, which allows for a 'medicinal' anthropology that goes beyond the mere description of ethnomedical practices. It helps us to understand people's search for health, and the shifts and transformations that arise from the movements and connections of people and things in the capitalist world economy.

References

Illich I (1976) *Limits to Medicine. Medical Nemesis: The Expropriation of Health*. Harmondsworth: Penguin.

Moerman D (2000) Cultural variations in the placebo effect: ulcers, anxiety and blood pressure. *Medical Anthropology Quarterly* 14: 51–72.

Nichter M (1996) Popular perceptions of medicine: a south Indian case study, in Nichter M and Nichter M (eds) *Anthropology and International Health. Asian Case Studies*. Amsterdam: Gordon & Breach 203–37.

Turner V (1967) *The Forest of Symbols. Aspects of Ndembu Ritual*. Ithaca, London: Cornell University Press.

Van der Geest S and Whyte SR (1989) The charm of medicines: metaphors and metonyms. *Medical Anthropology Quarterly* 3: 345–67.

Whyte SR, Van der Geest S and Hardon A (2002) *Social Lives of Medicines*. Cambridge: Cambridge University Press.

9 Local and global medicines

Overview

The aim of this chapter is to explore the mobility of medicines and the transform-ations of meanings and social practices, that their movements can entail. As we mentioned at the end of the previous chapter, medicines with different origins and with ideas attached to them move and are given new meanings in the social and cultural contexts they enter. Under conditions of a global capitalist market, drugs and ideas about them are distributed everywhere by the marketing efforts of pharmaceutical companies, within reach of all who can pay for them. In turn, local medicines, such as herbs, enter global circuits through the growing interest of these companies and new 'alternative' medical practitioners, scientists and consumers. In this chapter, we shall look at some of the many movements of medicines between different social, cultural and economic contexts, and at the effects of these movements: how syringes move from biomedical institutions into African villages; how herbal medicines move from the bush into scientific laboratories; and how anti retroviral (ARV) drugs move from global market into local sufferers' families.

Learning objectives

By the end of this chapter you should have gained some insight into:

- **the indigenization of a biomedical object into new contexts**
- **the appropriation of non-biomedical medicines into a scientific pharmaceutical frame**
- **the place of medicines in the capitalist world economy**
- **the complex social effects of ARV medication in HIV high-prevalence populations**

Key terms

Commodification Process in which things in people's lives are replaced by commodities, objects that are produced for the purpose of exchange and considered to contain an inherent value that can be translated into the equivalent of another commodity or a monetary exchange medium. Commodification is linked to the replacement of gift economies, in which things derive their value explicitly from social relations, by commodity economies.

Generic drugs The basic active component of a pharmaceutical, irrespective of who produced it, in contrast to a branded drug, which is produced and often patented by a particular company. Generic drugs are usually the cheaper alternative to branded drugs.

Indigenization This term usually applies to the process of adaptation to the local social and cultural environment that Western biomedicine undergoes when it becomes part of non-Western medical systems. However, it could also refer to the inclusion of aspects of non-Western medical traditions into biomedicine (for example acupuncture).

Modern A concept ordering the world by opposing itself to what belongs to the past: tradition. A narrative device that organizes time, space and social differences around the fiction of a great leap forward in history – the gap between those who made the leap and those who did not (yet) do so and remain 'traditional'.

Traditional Used in opposition to 'modern', with connotations of local (versus global or universal), static (versus dynamic), of the past (versus of today and the future). There is no 'tradition' without 'modernity', and vice versa as both concepts are mutually constituted.

The appropriation of syringe and needle

The relationship between biomedicine and non-biomedical realms of medical practice can imply a movement of medicines or techniques from biomedicine into other social contexts; this process has been called (with an involuntary derogatory slant) 'indigenization' of pharmaceuticals (Bledsoe and Goubaud 1985). For example, fishermen in western Kenya commonly sprinkled the content of antibiotic capsules on infected wounds, which improved their condition but deviated from biomedical practice. In the same villages, the priestesses of an African independent Church, *Legio Maria*, at times dressed like hospital nurses, referred to their Holy Water as 'our procaine penicillin' and gave infants 'injections with the cross' to protect them from sickness, innovating both medicine and Christian ritual (Prince 1999). In the same area, some healers encouraged patients to bring their x-rays to divination sessions to improve their diagnosis.

Medicines are indigenized everywhere in the world, not only in Africa. Driven by mistrust in the medical profession and science, in the West, especially where public health services are insufficient, such as in the USA, people rely increasingly on the Internet to shop for medicines as well as for medical information, which is often at variance with established biomedical views and which frequently includes other, 'exotic' medical treatments. Similarly driven by mistrust in faltering government health provision as well as by lack of law enforcement and by aggressive drug marketing, people in developing countries rely on pharmaceuticals bought from shops or exchanged between neighbours.

For many people, hypodermic needles and syringes epitomize biomedical treatment. Being painful, injections are feared, but at the same time they are desired because they are believed to be powerful. In some settings where the public health system has deteriorated together with an increase in HIV prevalence, people have lost their trust in government health provision, and have come to fear hospitals as places where one loses money, gets few and inefficient medicines, and might even become infected with HIV. In response to this distrust in official medicine – biomedical knowledge and power – people have appropriated, literally, the key medicines, syringes and injections, and privatized or domesticated them. For example, many households in western Kenya possess their own syringes and injectables, many fathers inject their own families, and many people prefer private and local, often untrained, injectionists to government health facilities (see Birungi, 1998, for similar findings in Uganda). Having one's own syringes does not only afford protection from the dangers of official medical institutions; it positively affirms responsibility and agency, by making the father into the primary provider of life-sustaining medicine for his children, for example. In this way, people effectively get rid of *medicine* – institutions, doctors and professional knowledge – and retain the *medicines*: mobile objects of healing, powerful tools and tokens of autonomy and agency.

Moreover, inserting biomedical techniques and drugs into familiar relations merges their material potency with that of personal caring relations, ensuring and reinforcing the effects; as Birungi (1998) writes, concerning 'domesticized' injections in Uganda:

> To be sure of the quality of treatment people obtain injections from someone they already know and make decisions of where to seek treatment after consulting neighbours, family and colleagues . . . Getting treatment from a person well known to the user instils confidence in the correctness of the medicine and the safety of the injection . . . 'You can be sure when the injection is provided by a person you know' . . . Social relations do not only guarantee protection and support to the patient, but also serve as a means of gaining access to a symbolic token of healing. When a family member proposed to a patient with severe hernia pains to be taken to a nearby government hospital to undergo a surgical operation . . . another family member asked: 'You are suggesting that we take him to hospital. Do you know anybody working there?'

The power of local social bonds and the power of substances should shape and enable each other. Good medicines should have a place in good relations.

From a public health perspective, one problem of indigenization is that medicines, absorbed into local context and disconnected from the doctor–patient relationship, are often used in unintended ways, for example overdosing and underdosing, taking too many different medicines, or too short courses of drugs. Medical anthropologists in public health can contribute to the solution of such problems by pointing the health worker beyond the simplified solutions such as health education and drug control, important as these remain. If rational drug use is to be promoted then it is first necessary to understand the rationalities that appear at variance with the biomedical one.

The appropriation of traditional medicine

The relation between biomedicine and non-biomedical practices can also move in the opposite direction, when supposedly traditional medicines are carried into 'modern' frames dominated by biomedicine, science or market economy. We shall look at this process, using the example of African 'traditional' herbal medicine.

In the beginning of colonial occupation, the European occupiers were interested in African, herbal medical solutions to the deadly threats to which biomedicine as yet knew no answer. After the late nineteenth-century attitudes changed due to the victory of germ theory in European medicine and missionary resentment of the link between African herbs and ancestral religion. African healers became 'witchdoctors', symbols of 'backwardness', enemies of colonial modernity. In recent decades this rejection has been partly reversed. This began, after formal independence from colonial occupation, with the rediscovery of African 'heritage', which led to the formation, in many African nations, of professional bodies of traditional healers, analogous to biomedical bodies with their bureaucratic institutions, written codices and certificates of expertise – the professionalization of African medicine (Last and Chavunduka 1986). The designation of particular practices and ideas as 'traditional' implies modern thinking, so the state endorsement of traditional medicine implied changes to its knowledge and practice. New organizations were often male dominated, herbal medicines became more important than rituals and social relations, concerns with dosage and timing of medication were based on the biomedical model, and the idea of a coherent expert medical knowledge replaced the more democratic and eclectic use of herbs within families and villages, with prepacked remedies from herbal 'doctors' sometimes replacing herbs from the bush or garden (see Figure 9.1).

Subsequently, governments and aid organizations began to include healers in public health interventions, particularly related to HIV/AIDS. There have been reports about some positive results, but it is important to examine the wider effects of such intervention. By designating some healers and not others as suitable collaborators, by giving them formal training and informal learning experiences, and by structuring the collaboration along the lines of public health institutions and international donor cashflows, the category of traditional healer is recreated in a process that should be studied instead of being taken for granted.

Parallel with the renewed appreciation of healers, the potential usefulness of herbal medicines to identify new pharmaceutical compounds was recognized. This raises political and economic questions such as the problem of intellectual property rights, especially when private companies are involved. A widespread view is that bioprospecting drug companies should give something back to the original owners of the herbs, which raises the question, who these owners are – local people, traditional healers, governments, landowners? – and what a fair share of the profits would be. The newly evoked global relations through which herbal medicines move provide a complex field for anthropological studies (see e.g. Hayden 2003).

One approach to these complexities is to follow the herbal medicine on its journey, asking what happens to herbs and herbal knowledge on the way from the house of an African mother to the pharmaceutical laboratory (and into a marketable drug, which might eventually be sold back to the African mother). On its way, the medicine is collected from the thicket, extracted, literally from the forest and from the plant itself, and metaphorically, from social relations, beliefs and rituals, and isolated. Then it is resocialized in clinical trials and legal processes up to its licensing as a drug. Apart from issues of power, ownership and justice, the anthropologist is interested in what is lost in this translation and what is gained. Moreover, attention to the transformations of the medicine along this way allows us to learn about the specificity of scientific and biomedical notions of substance, potency, healing and the body. The following description of ethnobotanical research in Kenya illustrates this.

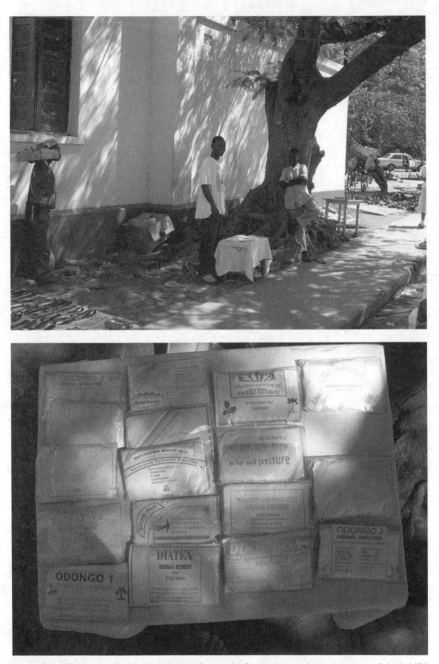

Figure 9.1 'Traditional' herbal medicines for viral infections on sale in an area with high HIV prevalence, western Kenya 2004 (photographs Wenzel Geissler (not previously published))

Activity 9.1

Read the excerpt below from the paper 'Persons and relations in the work of ethno-botanical knowledge' by Geissler and Prince (n.d.), bearing in mind the following questions:

1 What is lost during the journey of herbal medicines described here? How could that affect the usefulness of the research?
2 Which characteristics of the scientific or biomedical approach to disease can be identified in this (partial) re-creation of a herbal remedy as a pharmaceutical?

Collections, identifications and extracts

Herbaria

During the last months of fieldwork, we gathered about a hundred medicinal plant specimens, dried them between newspaper leaves, and carried them home to Europe. The most beautiful of these consisted of leaves, flowers and fruits or of whole plants in flower and their fruits, gathering the plant's different life-stages into a single object.

This collection had its difficulties: to obtain a complete sample depended upon the season, and required collection of specimen from the same plant at different times; different women's knowledge was at variance with one another, the same plants were given different names and the same names used for different plants, the same plant was used for different illnesses and prepared differently by different women; illnesses were often impossible to translate, and their signs diffuse; some plants were used but had no name, other were given names and attributed power, but the women did not know for what. Many of these problems were solved by the method: each time a woman pointed at a plant, we asked for the name, the illness it treated, and the part used and the preparation. Mixtures were recorded by cross-reference on each of the plants. If a plant had several uses, we used several sheets, so that each sheet eventually came to stand for one 'medicine'. Information that did not fit into this schema was simply omitted.

We found expert help to 'identify' the plants, that is to ascribe to them Latin names and the place in the Linnaean classification scheme, in the Oxford University Herbarium. Here specimens were carefully removed from the Kenyan newspapers and attached to thick, white sheets of paper with small paper strips and glue. The sheets were numbered, and after identification, small labels were tied to the plants, and the sheets were stored, according to their place in the botanical classification, in one of the drawers of the large and old herbarium. Information on uses and identifications were assembled in a database, and earlier ethnobotanical findings were added for comparison; this table was subsequently published in an ethnobotanical journal. By a few dramatic transformations and geographical dislocations, the same plant had been removed from the undifferentiated, impenetrable bush, made into a specimen, and re-inserted into a highly differentiated, two-dimensional and unequivocal botanical and archival system. Some relations were lost, but others were gained in this process.

Laboratories

Once this information was available, our colleagues in medical parasitology wondered whether these plants were 'effective' against parasites such as worms or malaria and set out to answer this question by testing the plants' effect against various worms and microbes. For the production of the plant extracts used in this in vitro screening (observing the effect of plant extract on organisms in a glass tube), large amounts of plant material were collected and '250 mg of plant powder were weighed into a test tube and mixed with 2.5 ml extraction fluid in an ultrasound bath for two hours. The test tube was left in a refrigerator over night. In the morning the extract was centrifuged at 2–3000 rounds per minute for 5 minutes. The supertenant was transferred into a beaker. Where the supertenant was turbid, the extract was passed through a filter dipped into extraction fluid. These raw extracts were used for the screening of the plant material against micro-organisms' (all quotes from Olsen and Nielsen 1999). Here, the plant's pure capacity was almost reached.

But not yet quite. The extracts were employed in 'bioassays' testing their activity against a range of organisms. For the bacteria and fungi, 'bioautography' was employed: spots of plant extract were placed on petri dishes with a growth medium, then the dishes were sprayed with the organisms in question; after inoculation, the dishes were sealed with sterile film and incubated at body temperature; after incubation and further chemical treatment, one could discern 'inhibition zones' around the plant extract spots, which indicate the plant extract's capacity to delimit growth or, ideally, to extinguish the organism. As the method's name indicates, life, or the capacity to prevent it, inscribes itself on the surface of the artificial growth medium. For the blood parasites, human blood, infected with the parasites was incubated for two days with the plant extracts, a radioactive medium was added, and after drying the parasites, their rate of growth or proliferation was measured. The outcome was growth inhibition, with the ideal of 100%, equaling complete eradication. As for the worms, they were exposed to the plant extracts in a series of concentrations, and after respectively one hour and one day's incubation, the worms were dyed to distinguish dead and living worms, and the percentage of dead ones was calculated to judge the effectiveness of the extract. While for the micro-organisms, 'growth inhibition' was the evaluation criterion, for the larger parasites, the ability to 'kill,' especially in low concentrations, was in focus. The main outcome measurement was 'the lowest effective concentration, which was able to kill all parasites in the medium'. In this standstill the definite truth, the pure capacity of the medical herb would have been revealed.

Based on the bioassays' results, the extract of one plant was chosen for a 'bioguided purification'. The plant extract was concentrated, freeze-dried, and run through a silica chromatography-column, which fractionated it, according to running speed, into 448 fractions, which by another chromatography method could be grouped into 18 fractions. When these again were tested bioautographically, two were particularly 'active' against fungi. These were concentrated and freeze-dried, diluted and run through a different column-chromatography which split it into 22 fractions, of which four proved active and were again dried, diluted and fractionated in a third column, providing 185 fractions, of which two active ones were selected for further structural analysis. A concentration of 25 μg completely stopped the growth of the fungus. In a concentration of 0.08 mg/ml the same substance could kill parasites. Unfortunately the substance had been purified in insufficient amounts to clarify its structure through NMR spectroscopy'.

When the latter was attempted, 'possible signals from the active substance A had disappeared in the background noise'. The other substance, B, underwent the same test but it 'had undergone a chemical transformation during the cleaning process' and was 'insufficiently purified' to read the atoms' signals clearly. The limits of purification were reached.

This is where our study of Uhero's plants ended. The aim of this search was finality; the atoms, purified from distractions and changes, standing still and emitting their true signals. Truth as the end of time and process. We almost reached it, but as often in scientific research, a little way remained.

Ethnopharmacology: from village kitchen to the atom's signals

This summary of our study has shown some of the effort to make Kenyan medicines known: this work could be described as a series of movements of extraction, separation, purification from the entanglements of thick thornbush and women's talk, beliefs and everyday lives, through herbaria and test tubes, to the atoms of the 'active principle'; a search for essence, in which substance and capacity fall in one, without need for further reference or relation.

In the first parts of this process, the work extracts the herb from its various contexts, from the relations to people, soil and seasons, and concentrates the plant medicine as a whole into one, named thing; this is achieved when the herbarium sheet containing all the plant's life-stages is labelled with its Latin name, uses and preparation, and positioned within the cupboards of the Oxford Herbarium; in this age-old collection the plant is released from place and time; all its original strings have been dissolved and translated into the notes on the edges of the white cardboard. The second part of the process follows an opposite strategy, progressively splitting up the carefully constituted whole plant – grinding, extracting, fractionating etc. – down to its, in this context indivisible, atoms. The peculiar criterion of separation in this narrowing gaze is whether the substance can prevent life or kill, or not, and how little substance is needed to achieve this goal. The plant's potential capacity to restore the human body is thus gauged by its ability to kill that which is adverse to it, within a logic of irreconcilable animosity between individual bodies and equally individual parasites.

While separation and purification, disentanglement from relations between the substance of capacity and others – plants, persons, substances – are the stated goals of each of the many transformations that this scientific endeavour engages even in this abridged account it is clear that at every stage new connections are made. Take the Herbarium: not only are there relations of people, and of specimens in the classification and shelving, and of past and present researchers through the cross-referencing and comparison of evidence, there is also the past in a much wider sense that the University and its collections embody, and a future for which this particular institution accumulates and preserves plants and knowledge. Or take the last stage of the laboratory work: the groups of scientists working on different diseases all over the world, the experts on animal models, the laboratory animals, worms and microbes, the spectrophotometers, the chromatography systems; and, looming in the future, pharmaceutical companies, pipelines of synthetic production, and trials on human populations, which potentially would take the extracted, purified, identified and synthesised active substance back to the people of places like Kenya, to test the efficacy and safety of new drugs. Thus, in this process, ostensibly of purification and isolation, new worlds are opened, new fields of 'activity' for the Kenyan herbs conquered, and ever-widening networks of connections woven.

The original webs of relatedness in local kinship and ritual ideas in which the herbs were used in the village are transformed and replaced by manifold and wide-ranging ramifications of new connections. What is changed is the scale of the networks in which capacity is sought and found, but not their complexity. One way of making the plants known is not more 'holistic' or 'reductionist' than the other. The difference could rather be said to lie in how the relationship between separations and relations is constituted. For the scientist, the separated, stable state of an entity is its 'nature', which purification and splitting up aim to identify; relations are here secondary to the primary identity of the entity in question.

The cited research reports present a trajectory to the bottom of matter, which apparently simply is there. Yet, the methodological efforts and problems the reports describe show that this 'essence' is man-made, an act of creativity and work, and despite the tremendous transformations that indeed have been achieved from village kitchens to the chromatography column, no end has been reached. Scientists would conceptualize the problems in the interaction between human and non-human in this play of discovery as a left-over, a margin of error, a lack of precision that will be remedied by ever sharper tools. As long as we can make things purer, we move towards truth. This foregrounding of separation is where the scientists' engagement with the plants differs from the villagers': for them, the plant's erratic collaboration in medicinal treatment is part of an unpredictable relationship between plant and human; many of these relations are given names, such as spirits, the ancestors, the earth; for the villagers, these other movements are not leftovers on the way to pure knowledge and capacity: they are the source of capacity, which one needs to continuously engage with in order to maintain health and well-being.

↻ Feedback

1 Some information is lost, such as information about mixtures of herbs, which may be vital for their pharmacological effect. More importantly, social relations and cultural knowledge of herb use are erased; some herbs may be linked to rituals, others to faith, which could influence their medicinal effects and the sufferers' experience of these. The potency of medicine is examined only in terms of chemical effects upon physical bodies, which might be a reason why few similar bio-assay based ethnobotanical studies successfully identify new pharmacological compounds.

2 The restricted notion of sickness as disease, which is rooted in the body and can be uprooted by chemical means; the emphasis on disease-agents or germs, which have to be fought to restore health; the aim of eradicating germs and purifying the body; the idea that capacity lies within entities, such as molecules, rather than in relations between people and substances; the notion that truth is to be revealed by isolation and purification of principles, and by reproducible, context-free experiments.

The movements of medicines through the global market

Irrespective of whether they are based on laboratory synthesis or on African herbs, when medicines are industrially produced and exchanged within capitalist regimes they become commodities. This entails that they are not primarily embedded in social relations – like herbal remedies within a family or community, for example – but things-in-themselves. As objects of market exchange, they can be detached from producers or owners because payment, at least in principle, relinquishes the exchange relation. They can subsequently leave the commodity sphere and become gifts or tokens of affection, but their origin as commodities, free from immediate social links but tied to monetary exchanges, distinguishes them.

One peculiar trait of commodified pharmaceuticals is that not only are the medicines produced industrially but the knowledge about them is also produced and controlled centrally through advertising and public relations strategies. Moreover, the flow of knowledge is more-or-less in one direction – from companies to consumers.

This raises the anthropological question of how supposedly passive consumers deal with the information that they are offered, and what effects marketing and advertising has. Thus, it has been shown in the Philippines that advertisements for common medicines not only influence consumer behaviour and drug consumption but also ideas of illness and its causes. Moreover, the drug advertisements did not only relate information on the drugs themselves but also played on and used gender relations, family ideals and values of maternal responsibility in the target communities (Tan 1999). Thus, advertisements, far from simply helping people to use the right medicines, linked people's social life and culture, their notions of illness and wellbeing, and the interest of the company and its owners, around particular pharmaceuticals.

The same applies to branding. In western Kenya, different brand names of identical antimalarial drugs influenced their use. For example, an antimalarial, which the drug company had called Homaquin, because coastal Kenyans often refer to malaria symptoms as *homa*, was in western Kenya deemed 'weak', compared to chloroquine, because there the term *homa* is applied to flu and cold-like symptoms; it was ranked as equally ???? as 'Homanol', a local brand of paracetamol (Prince *et al.* 2001).

Such marketing issues can be of relevance to public health intervention. For example, when many African nations changed their recommended first-line malaria treatment from chloroquine to sulphadoxine-pyrimethamine (SP), the ways in which this change was promoted, in conjunction with particular political situations and people's relations with the government, played a key role in how the transition was received. Thus, in north-western Tanzania, many people were suspicious of government antimalarial drug policies as part of widespread suspicions about corruption and 'business interests' in the context of a newly 'liberalized' or privatized capitalist economy (Soori Nnko personal communication). Instead of assuming that government public health provides good medicine, the assumption was that politics and business were inseparable in the contemporary world. Anti-retroviral treatment for HIV/AIDS is another politicized example of the changing relations between pharmaceuticals, the market, sick people and others.

The challenge of antiretroviral treatment and HIV

Pharmaceuticals often aim at finishing disease and curing the patient by eliminating the disease agent, as exemplified by anti-infectious drugs, epitomizing the power of biomedicine. This idea of pharmaceuticals as single magic-bullet solutions that can eradicate disease has been challenged by HIV/AIDS. Although this is a biomedically defined infection, the 'germ' in question cannot be eradicated by a pharmaceutical. Anti-retroviral drugs (ARVs) are not just bought, ingested and forgotten like antibiotics: one's life becomes dependent upon them, days are restructured, habits are changed, and relations to other people are reshaped. In populations with high HIV prevalence, such changes affect the whole social order and its cultural values.

Activity 9.2

Read the abridged article from Whyte et al. (2004) below, keeping in mind the following questions:

1   What are the channels of ARV distribution and the role of government control?
2   Why could the introduction of ARVs in Uganda change social life and values despite the fact that few people have access to them?

Treating AIDS: dilemmas of unequal access in Uganda

Introduction
In the international media, differential access to AIDS medicine exemplifies global inequalities between wealthy and poor countries. Price cuts by multinational pharmaceutical companies, the advent of cheaper generics, action research programmes and donor support for treatment offer ways of remedying these inequities. Yet equal access to treatment is still a long way off. The drop in price has created dilemmas for a minority who could never have considered treatment at the old price, but who have just enough resources to make the cheaper drugs an almost realistic option. In this article, we explore these dilemmas, as people learn about options, make painful choices and imagine the possibilities open to others as well as themselves. Who should have the drugs and who can get them?

Our theme is that AIDS medicine is socially as well as pharmacologically active, in that it occasions reflections on social relations and distinctions. Health care workers and ordinary citizens are increasingly confronting the reality of unequal access. For some this is a matter of moral concern; for others it is the normal order of things; for others still, it is a practical problem with which to deal, or to overlook while tackling more immediate difficulties. Our ambition is not only to document pharmaceutical policy and inequality, but to show their significance for differently positioned Ugandans as they work out a vernacular view of social pharmacy.

The social lives of AIDS medicines
We set the scene by tracing the life courses of ARVs as they enter Uganda and flow through alternative channels to sick bodies. ARV drugs originate as branded products from five multinational pharmaceutical firms and as generics from several Indian companies. Under an initiative from UNAIDS, the multinationals set up an

autonomous organisation in 1999, Medical Access Uganda Limited, to ensure a steady supply of AIDS drugs to gazetted treatment centres, with a small profit margin to cover costs. When Indian companies entered the market with generics, they did not come in through this initiative, but set up distributorships at Kampala pharmacies. Two of the multinationals followed suit, establishing sales representatives dedicated to AIDS products at a Kampala retail outlet. In addition to the drugs imported through these established channels, others find their way from Europe through the hands of individuals who bring them in for themselves, friends or family, or perhaps to sell again. Once in the country, ARVs flow out to sick people through four kinds of more or less well-demarcated channels.

One way in which they are made available is through treatment and research programmes, funded by donors and provided for free. These projects can in 2003 only provide treatment for a few thousand people, and are localised and have strict eligibility requirements. Mainly branded drugs from the big multinationals flow to these projects. Because they are donor funded, supply is ensured for the life of the project at least, and there is fairly good control over the provision of the treatment. A second channel provides drugs to gazetted treatment centres. Most of these are fee-for-service, although some free drugs are provided through research studies. While the donor research and treatment programmes and the gazetted treatment centres are not government financed, they are very much government approved and have a public character and presence. They have a professional character of the type that contributes to what a recent article in the *Lancet* called 'Preventing antiretroviral anarchy in sub-Saharan Africa'. The third channel, private practitioners, is far more discreet and less open to surveillance. No one knows exactly how many private physicians are treating patients with ARVs. Once someone has a prescription, it is possible to have it filled without continuously consulting a doctor – this opens the door for more creative and less systematic use of medicine. The fourth channel is hardly a channel at all, but a web of capillaries through which ARVs seep out to those in need. People who are 'in the system' help relatives and friends to obtain the drugs at lowest possible cost. Whether anarchy, or at least disorder that is convenient for some, will set in remains to be seen. Will ARVs be diverted from their enclaved positions under the monopoly of health professionals in quasi-public institutions? Such valuable commodities, needed desperately in a poor country where people look for any way to make money, will provide a strong challenge to the kind of structured framework called for by the authors of the *Lancet* article.

Inclusion criteria: what about me?

These channels distribute ARVs unequally. Official channels apply inclusion criteria, as funds are scarce. A prime example is a programme to prevent mother-to-child transmission. Mothers who attended antenatal clinics are counselled about the possibility of receiving a free dose of the ARV nevirapine at onset of labour, and a dose for the newborn baby, which can reduce vertical transmission by about 50%. Mothers wishing to participate must take an HIV test; the medicine is only given to those who test positive. It can save the baby but has no effect upon the mother, for whom no treatment is offered. This requires women to confront distressing information, which will be made known to hospital staff, with differential consequences for themselves and the child. Social pharmacy cuts across the most intimate of all relations – that between mother and child. The ARV is for the baby; the mother can only lick the free milk powder that was also intended for the child.

The inequality of access to free therapy is illustrated by recent developments within The AIDS Support Organisation (TASO). In 2002, TASO decided to subsidise ARV treatment for its counsellors, introducing a deep distinction in the commonality of experience that the success of TASO rests on. Most clients of TASO have no chance of obtaining the same treatment. Donor-funded research and treatment projects have linked up with TASO to provide medicines and clinical care to clients who meet established criteria. The US medical research body, Communicable Disease Centre (CDC) have recruited the first 32 of a planned 1000 adults for a 3-year study (ARV treatment is promised for life for study subjects, but is not yet funded beyond the study period). The researchers have thought carefully about inclusion criteria: membership of TASO, CD4 count under 250; sleeping seven days a week in the surveyed household. Priority for admission to the study will go to those still surviving from a previous CDC study, then to members of the TASO Drama Club, and then chronologically in order of length of membership – those who joined TASO first get first chance. What is unclear is the effect this will have on those who are not part of the study. Part of the plan is to provide public education about ARVs. Awareness of ARVs will be raised. Yet most HIV-positive people in the district are not members of TASO; not even all of TASO's 7000–8000 members will be given drugs; and not even all sexual partners of the study subjects can be included. The question 'what about me?' is bound to arise as the project takes shape. Welcome as this project is, it shares with other donor-funded treatment initiatives a limited lifespan and access criteria that exclude many people. They are left to the 'public–private mix-up' that constitutes health care obtained from government facilities, fee-for-service clinics and retail drug outlets.

Painful priorities in families: affording the next dose

Ugandan families are large, and as every Ugandan knows, part of the practice of relatedness is giving and receiving assistance. People of all economic backgrounds depend on family help in dealing with illness. AIDS is different because of its long duration and the fact that it often strikes more than one person in a family. Families with a member needing ARVs have already been burdened by caring for long and demanding illnesses, and possibly by the cost of funeral expenses and fostering orphans. Only families with relatively good resources consider undertaking costly and lifelong treatment with ARVs. Even for them, the burden is often too heavy . . .

Treating AIDS means withdrawing support to other relatives for other important life projects. Patients reported that it was not easy for them to decide stopping or reducing financial support for relatives because extended families, fictive kinship institutions, neighbours, and close friends were social assets, and were always mobilised or united when a disaster struck. So there was a fear that they would also lose such support in the future. People speculate about whether taking a child out of school would enable them to buy drugs and improve enough to keep a job so they could continue giving at least some support. They worry about using all their resources to buy drugs, not being able to continue after they run out of money and then dying, leaving their children with nothing. The price of social relations and life chances is brought sharply to consciousness in such situations.

Because more than one family member is often sick, treating AIDS means choosing whom to help. Sometimes families do pull together and find enough resources for all, at least for a while. George and Lisa wed in 1990 and had been blessed with three children. When their last-born child fell ill, failed to respond to treatment, and died in 2000, they could hardly grasp the tragedy and the terrible thoughts for the future of the family. When they tested for HIV, both George and Lisa and their second born were HIV-positive. George worked for one of the most powerful companies in Kampala and was doing well. Although he was from a prosperous family and had close relatives living outside Uganda, he was stressed, afraid of losing his job, and fearful that other people would learn about his HIV status. He and Lisa both started using ARVs, but he still kept his diagnosis a secret until his financial status was in jeopardy. He lost the good job and the family depended on Lisa's income. In 2002, George fell ill with signs and symptoms of AIDS; his condition was no more a secret. It was rumoured that both George and Lisa had stopped using ARVs because they could no longer afford them. At this point family meetings were organised every Sunday by George's family, later involving Lisa's relatives as well. Resolutions to fundraise and purchase ARVs for all three were passed, medical check ups were done, and George improved enough to get another job. The financial and emotional costs of treating AIDS force people to conceptualise and make explicit assumptions about relationships that usually remain implicit. George and Lisa's relatives formalised this process through weekly meetings. Our colleague Mary explains how her family network financed one of her cousins' ARV treatment for a period when the cousin was very sick. Now the cousin has recovered, is working as a tailor, and is paying for her own treatment. 'It's a miracle,' Mary says. 'She was dying and now she is even paying school fees for her children.' Another member of the family is also HIV positive and in need of ARV treatment, but she has not managed to mobilise resources from the family network. Mary remarks: 'That one – she is not responsible, she doesn't understand ARV medicine, she never finished school and doesn't have a job. How do you start to help a person like this? People have to prioritise their resources: Do you pay ARV medicine for a sister forever and give up paying school fees for your child?' Mary is weighing up not just her relationships to her cousins, but their characters and their likelihood of resuming responsibilities within the family.

People who are ill and unable to support themselves must consider the burden that ARV therapy might impose upon their families. From the point of view of the sick person, being so highly dependent is often a distressing situation. Papa M is a retired government official, a wealthy and well-educated man by local standards. Three of his daughters knew that they had been infected with HIV. One died in 1998, before less expensive ARV medicine was available in Uganda. Another daughter, Prisca, started to lose weight after her husband died in 2000. When we discussed the cost of ARV treatment, Papa said: 'Even if we can't afford this in the long run we have to try it – we have to try it. She might pick up and survive. If she dies we will know that we tried everything possible.' She moved back to her parents' home, and her father and some of her brothers and sisters were buying the ARV drugs every month. Papa mobilised funds from daughters and sons for their sick sister, but most of them were incapable of helping in a significant way, having many children themselves for whom to care. When a third daughter Lovisa, who had moved in to help care for sister Prisca, fell sick, she decided not to stay at home: 'It is too hard for mother to see our sister Prisca being sick. It reminds her of how our other sister died . . . The medicine helps, but it puts pressure on mother. She worries about how they will get the next dose, money, transport . . . So I decided to move where she can't see me and worry about me.' Meanwhile, Prisca had many side-effects from the medication. Papa M said that he suspected she lost the morale to take the drugs. She died on Easter Sunday. The family was again in great pain, and Papa commented that it was depressing to have spent so much money and put great expectations in these new drugs, which proved to be worthless for his daughter.

He did not talk about the third daughter who is also HIV-positive, but from his facial expressions it was clear that his worries continued. Lovisa's sensitivity about being a burden to her family increased accordingly.

These family situations do not involve priority setting once and for all, but rather continuing processes unfolding over time as circumstances change and one set of problems overshadows another. When a relative is desperately ill, it is usually possible to mobilise help. But after the first few months on ARVs, if the patient improves, the family again feels the weight of other obligations and stops contributing to purchasing the drugs. The long-term commitment to buying ARVs is difficult for individuals and families to maintain in situations where needs are so abundant. The medical consequences of these family dilemmas are non-adherence to treatment regimens and the 'antiretroviral anarchy,' with dangers of developing resistance, that experts fear. Health workers regularly confront the realities of patients not being able to pay for treatment, and families who have some means struggling to balance the cost of the next dose against all the other needs. At the same time, we found a recurring conviction that well-placed people could afford them or get them through connections.

Connections, secrecy and status: those big people

We often heard people say: 'those big people get medicines to prolong their lives'. Medicinal knowledge is social knowledge, or at least it is linked to people's image of the kind of society in which they live. But the political imagination about social status and access to medicine has one particular feature that is especially striking: the conviction that the elite takes medicines secretly. From one point of view, secrecy is simply understandable discretion and a desire for confidentiality, which also may be due to the fact that stigma increases with socio-economic status. Wealthy and well-connected people do not want to associate their symptoms with HIV or to disclose their status. Social differences mean that some people have more face to save than others.

Others put forward the view that secrecy is a political and moral issue. There are two issues here. One is the question of whether state money is being used clandestinely to favour the few. The other is the matter of the role of openness and solidarity in the fight against AIDS.

Leading AIDS activist Major Rubaramira told us that there were perhaps 1000 Ugandans who receive medicine from different government sources. 'But no one talks about it. These are all big people and getting medicine makes them support the government.' For Rubaramira, the misuse of public trust and public resources is not in itself so unexpected. Worse than the cheating are the hypocrisy and the secrecy which have become commonplace among HIV-positive elites. It is not so much that people resent wealth and advantage as such. What is objectionable is secret consumption and selfish unwillingness to affirm relations with others by sharing and helping. What is morally admirable, at least in the eyes of enlightened AIDS professionals, is the willingness to speak out and stand with others in the struggle against the disease. The views of people like Major Rubaramira harmonise with a deep theme in dealings with misfortune: the morality of open public affirmation of relationships and the ambiguity and potential evil of secret use of medicines for purely selfish ends. Just as medicines (both African and cosmopolitan) have the possibility of secret use in the local rural communities, so people imagine that ARVs can be taken without regard for sociality. As long as they are so expensive for ordinary people, the image of the powerful man getting them covertly through connections can only be a bitter one, and raises questions about morality.

Conclusion

ARVs have powerful symbolic potential. As concrete things, they objectify relationships in both subtle and dramatic ways. Hope, concern, solidarity, power, money, selfishness are all enacted as those tablets and capsules move between people. Access to ARVs in Uganda illustrates the social meanings of medicines with painful clarity. Research and treatment projects with their inclusion and exclusion criteria, families who have to choose which lives to support, and activists who call for social justice – all are caught up in dilemmas. As global pharmaceuticals, ARVs have captured the social and political imagination more powerfully than almost any other kind of medicine.

↻ Feedback

1 The four channels described are: (a) research and donor-funded programmes; (b) government treatment centres; (c) private practitioners and sales representatives; (d) friends and kin relations. The authors argue that the need for ARVs is such that state control will be defeated by cultural creativity and market forces. While this is supported by much of their research, one should be careful not to give up the crucial role of the state in the provision and control of pharmaceuticals. While it is difficult for the Ugandan government to control multinational drug companies or other well-endowed actors, bilateral or international government bodies should co-ordinate their efforts to govern ARV drug flows.

2 Anti retroviral drugs become symbols of survival in societies overwhelmed by the spectre of death. Their non-availability and the secrecy surrounding them enhance rather than diminish their potency to transform the social and political imaginary. In this context it is worth noting that people in East Africa already suspected white people of possessing, but withholding, AIDS cures in the early 1990s, before the advent of ARVs. Thus, these pharmaceuticals already served as a vehicle to critique power differentials before they existed. Beyond the embodiment of such negative, selfish and unequal relations, ARVs and their availability or otherwise can embody relations of responsibility, care and love. In this way they serve as a subject for ethical and political debates.

Summary

In this chapter we looked at what happens to medicines when they move between contexts with diverging kinds of knowledge and institutional order. It is not possible to judge whether such movements are desirable or not, as there is no 'right place' for a particular medicine. A popularized pharmaceutical might serve people's health or damage it, and an industrialized herbal remedy might benefit the communities it originated from as much as new users, or it may serve solely the profit of the company that patented it. For medical anthropology, the primary issue is not whether such transfers ought to happen, but why they happen, what comes from them, what collateral effects they have, and how public health might engage with them. Only based on such thorough understanding will we be able to deal politically with these processes.

The same applies to the movements and transformations of medicines as commodities. At present, the production of pharmaceuticals lies mostly in the hands of privately owned corporations, but this dominance of the market is not total – for example, many democratic societies retain the production of vaccines and certain drugs under public control. Whether pharmaceuticals are produced for profit or for the common good remains a political question. Medical anthropology should not be paralysed by the dominance of uncontrolled market forces, but contribute to understanding, looking beyond and transforming existing conditions, and support the promotion of 'rational' drug use, based upon the priorities not of the shareholders of pharmaceutical companies, but of public health.

References

Birungi H (1998) Injections and self-help: risk and trust in Ugandan health care. *Social Science and Medicine* 47: 1455–62.

Bledsoe CH and Goubaud MF (1985) The reinterpretation of western pharmaceuticals among the Mende of Sierra Leone. *Social Science and Medicine* 21: 275–82.

Fabian J (1983) *Time and the Other. How Anthropology Makes its Object.* New York: Columbia University Press.

Good B (1994) *Medicine, Rationality and Experience. An Anthropological Perspective.* Cambridge: Cambridge University Press.

Hayden C (2003) *When Nature Goes Public. The Making and Unmaking of Bioprospecting in Mexico.* Princeton: Princeton University Press.

Horton R (1967) African traditional thought and Western science. *Africa* 37: 50–71 and 155–87.

Last M and Chavunduka G (eds) (1986) *The Professionalisation of African Medicine.* Manchester: Manchester University Press.

Olsen A and Nielsen B (1999) Undersøgelser af Lægeplanter benyttet af Luo folket i Kenya. MSc thesis, Institute for Medical Chemistry, University of Copenhagen.

Prince RJ (1999) The Legio Maria church in western Kenya: healing with the Holy Spirit and the rejection of medicines. MSc dissertation, Department of Anthropology, University College London.

Prince, RJ, Geissler, PW, Nokes, K *et al.* (2001) Knowledge of herbal and pharmaceutical medicines among Luo children in western Kenya. *Anthropology and Medicine* 8: 211–35.

Prince,RJ & Geissler PW (n.d.) Persons and relations in the work of ethnobotanical knowledge. Unpublished manuscript.

Tan M (1999) *Good Medicines: Pharmaceuticals and the Construction of Power and Knowledge in the Philippines.* Amsterdam: Het Spinhuis.

Whyte SR, Whyte MA, Meinert L and Kyaddondo B (2004) Treating AIDS: dilemmas of unequal access in Uganda. *Journal of Social Aspects of HIV/AIDS* 1: 14–26.

10 Cultures, persons, bodies

Overview

In this chapter we introduce the anthropological concept of personhood, which entails that persons, rather than being entities that are given, can be imagined and constructed differently. We argue that the notion of the individual as an indivisible and autonomous whole, with its own separate mind and body, which is at the centre of Western common sense and biomedicine, should be regarded as a cultural construct, which exists alongside, sometimes in conflict with, constructs of persons that are less focused on the idea of a unitary, independent entity and allow for a greater role of others in the production of the person. Different ideas of personhood and relatedness lead to different knowledges of the body and different bodily experiences and practices. In individualism, a notion of both person and body as bounded units goes along with a clear distinction between the body, matter, and the person, mind (see also Chapter 7). In the healthy person, the latter rules the former. Care for the body entails the maintenance of body limits and of self-control. If one instead regards the substantial, bodily relations that humans engage in – sharing food or place, sleeping with each other, kinship, working together – as the basis of personhood and of health, one de-emphasizes both the separateness of person and body, and the distinction between body and mind. From this, different approaches to the body and its wellbeing ensue. In this chapter, we will explore the relationship between personhood, body and health by studying different understandings of the person that do not primarily stress individuality. Furthermore, we shall look at interactions between cultural notions of personhood and changing socioeconomic conditions.

Learning objectives

By the end of this chapter, you should:

- understand the individual as one specific way of constructing personhood
- consider other concepts of personhood and their implications for the body and health
- understand the notion of *habitus* as analytical link between body, person and society
- become aware of how notions of personhood can conflict and change in one society
- appreciate the potential of bodily re-negotiations of power relations and personhood

Key terms

Dividual Used to capture the observation that among certain peoples and in particular situations, the person is understood not as individual but as extending into other persons and things, continuously divided and recomposed through social practices (see Strathern 1988).

Habitus Embodied dispositions that shape and delimit social practice; the concept helps to bridge between social structures outside the person and personal agency and will inside (Bourdieu 1977). Culture and society are inculcated as a habitus into bodies; persons are constrained as well as enabled by their habitus. For medical anthropology, the habitus is a tool to examine the interrelation of society, body and person in illness and health.

Hegemony The permeation throughout society of a system of values, attitudes, beliefs and so forth, that supports the status quo and becomes internalized to such an extent that it seems like common sense.

Individual Used here in the sense of a specific construct of the person that stresses autonomy, separateness, independence.

Possession States in which persons are displaced, subdued or struggling with spirits, who temporarily determine the body's actions, including speech.

Resistance Practices that challenge the exercise of domination through overt struggle or insidious forms of resilience (work evasion, sabotage, religious activity, drinking, or even sickness).

Sociality The practices that the people engage in to establish, maintain or dissolve, emphasize or hide, social relationships (different from society, which implies a bounded whole, constituted by an assembly of individual units that enter into relations).

Composite persons and bodies

Among the Luo of western Kenya, most people appreciate the contributions that other people and living and dead constituents of the environment make to the person. Sometimes, this acknowledgement of others' role is implicit in rules of hospitality and social intercourse. At other times it is explicitly spelled out; thus, some people consider ancestral and invisible personal forces as important parts of the person and adhere to ritual practices in their appreciation. In turn, many illnesses are attributed to disturbances of these vital links with others. Extending this notion of a <u>composite person</u>, which is open to external influences and relies upon them for wellbeing, many people think that worms and other physical agents are natural parts of the body and fulfil necessary functions (Geissler 1998; compare also the article by Nichter, Chapter 8). These internal agents can be harmful if provoked or occurring in excess, but they are not harmful as such.

Consequently, most treatment practices, especially for young children, aim at maintaining good relations with these agents and the environment: straightening or calming worms, responding to dead people's demands, shifting an illness to somebody else, or opening the body for flows of sweat, urine or faeces (Geissler and Prince 2005). This approach to treatment has, in relation to another East African society, been described by the anthropologist David Parkin (1995) as the 'dispersal' of sickness (as opposed to its 'eradication' as proposed by biomedicine, see below).

Healthy persons and bodies should be porous, continuous with their environment, rather than bounded. Medicines are used for the purpose of 'opening' the body or maintaining its natural openness towards others.

The Luo are not alone in holding such a view. In various other African societies, this notion of continuity or interfusion between persons, including invisible, dead, and absent persons and things that are regarded as persons, has been described as the basis of personhood and of notions of illness and treatment. In other societies, especially in south-east Asia and the western Pacific, exchanges of things (rather than flows) are considered to make persons. Thus some Melanesian peoples construct exchange objects such as pigs and shells as aspects of their persons, and in turn, they regard persons as 'partible', as able to detach parts of themselves in their interaction with others: a person can influence another through the 'part' that passes between them when, for example, a gift is exchanged (Strathern 1988). Even the person's gender is considered the product of human work and exchanges. Gender must thus be made and remade, rather than being biologically given at birth (as the Western notion of gendered, biological individuals suggests). In line with this place of things in relation to persons, exchange objects are critical to healing practices. Emphasizing the role of things in making persons from another angle, Indonesian ethnography has suggested that things, rather than being conceptualized simply as the possessions of individuals (as in the notion of personal property), are crucial to the construction of persons, relations and biographical narratives, and of wellbeing and sickness (Hoskins 1998). In turn, they are centrally involved in practices that maintain and restore bodily health.

These varied non-Western understandings of personhood have sometimes been described as 'dividuality', in order to emphasize the observer's experience of contrast *vis-à-vis* the more familiar notion of (originally) Western individualism. Individualism and dividuality appear in all societies, in varying proportions. They should not be reified as cultural essences and used to differentiate societies, such as in stereotypes of Western individualism versus African communalism, but should seen as tools to analyse and relate them. Even if certain peoples have an elaborate social imagination in which, for example, dividuality appears dominant, the same people live today in social worlds in which they position themselves towards more individual ideas and practices. And vice versa, even the most self-contained 'individualist' relies for his identity and well-being on relating with others. Cultural difference should therefore be sought within societies, among people that live together and engage with each other, not simply between societies. Moreover, such differences should not be taken as essential separations but should be explored as productive connections between cultures and societies.

For example, in the Kenyan Luo example that we started with, some people flatly reject the relational and open notion of person and body that we described, and emphasize individuality and hygiene, keeping themselves and their bodies apart from others. Often, this is linked to wider understandings of the person, for example in connection with faith or economic outlook, which do not only inform ideas about health but a wider worldview. Thus, some well-to-do, evangelical Christians feel equally threatened by germs, demons and distant, poorer relatives. For them, hygiene – for example avoiding a ritual meal honouring ancestors – can serve a medical, economic and moral purpose: it keeps the body protected, and marks the distinction from less well-to-do or from unchristian people. Most people in western Kenya manoeuvre between such diverging images of person and body, depending upon context and situation. They expect instant 'eradication' of sickness from a hospital medicine, but consult a diviner for the 'dispersal' of its true, relational, cause; they sterilize babies' bottles, but consider shared ritual meals indispensable for the children's health. Thus, we cannot say that the Luo, or other ethnic groups, adhere to a purely relational, or dividual, notion of the person (although they do give strong emphasis to social and bodily relations). The purpose of such designations is not to label, but to describe different aspects of social life.

For medical anthropologists in public health, categories like this help to maintain an awareness of diversity. Just as Luo ideas about worms are part of a wider culture of body and person, biomedicine is based upon a specific imagination of the person and is not simply the result of scientific discovery. Its own assumptions about the person as bounded, individual, autonomous, and split between ruling mind and ruled body, lead biomedicine to give preference to diseases that can be understood as boundary-infringements of individual bodies (such as infections), and to particular treatments that eradicate the agents of these diseases (germs), following a logic of warfare and exclusion. Therefore biomedicine is, although ubiquitous, not universally rooted in different places and social groups. The image of the modern, autonomous individual is omnipresent in our globally connected world, but it is just one possible image, emphasized to varying degrees in different times and places.

People's approaches to their bodies, health and illness rest upon different assumptions of what human beings are, which are tied in with faith, ethics and morality, and extend into all dimensions of everyday life. This means, for example, that bodily practices do not change as easily as health policy makers might wish, and given their broad implications, changing them depends upon wider societal changes and has wider consequences on society. Returning to our Luo example, the notion of the composite body and person implies that people aim at a good life with the potential of sickness they harbour, not at its eradication. Regarding child health, women say: 'a young child must be sick' (lest it may eventually die of an illness). This does not mean that people never take antibiotics or worm medicine but they are often taken in a slightly different way from the biomedical prescription: since the assumption is that the illness will stay with one anyway, one takes a little bit, whenever the illness reveals itself. While such 'irrational' drug use causes biomedical problems, it is rational under the given assumptions about the person.

Culture, person and bodily practice

Anthropology can help public health workers to understand other peoples' ways of dealing with their bodies and each other, based on knowledge of their social life and moral imagination. The problem that HIV/AIDS campaigns in Africa have to convince people of the usefulness of condoms can serve as an example. Christopher Taylor's ethnography of Rwandan notions of body and person and of economic change suggests that, with the introduction of capitalism in Rwanda, a new imaginary of the body and bodily wellbeing based on the ideal of containment and accumulation came to oppose an older image of the body as open to flows, and of health being predicated upon this openness (Taylor 1992). In one way of thinking about health, blockage meant illness and treatment meant opening, whereas in the other, closure equalled health and porosity sickness. Taylor goes on to argue that this conflictual constellation has implications for the epidemic of HIV/AIDS and the acceptance of condoms, and shows that even technical health interventions like condoms are embedded in complex and inert assumptions about body and person.

✎ Activity 10.1

Read the abridged article by Christopher Taylor (1990) below, keeping in mind the following questions:

1 What is the 'fractal person'?
2 How does the notion of the fractal person influence condom uptake?
3 Which implications for public health could be drawn from these insights?

📖 Condoms and cosmology: the 'fractal' person and sexual risk in Rwanda

Introduction

Recent studies reported that out of over 1000 sexually active adults in the Rwandan city of Kigali, 97% were reported to be aware that AIDS can be sexually transmitted. 71% reported serious concern about contracting AIDS, while only 17% claimed to have no fear of the disease. 58% of the people surveyed maintained that their anxiety about AIDS had led them to modify their sexual practices: 66% of the males were now avoiding casual contacts and contacts with prostitutes; 71% of the females had begun practicing abstinence or fidelity. Despite this evidence of growing Rwandan awareness about sexual practices and their impact upon AIDS transmission, none of the study's respondents reported the use of condoms during intercourse. While 69% of the men and 47% of the women knew what a condom was, among the women, 59% claimed that they did not like condoms. It is not the intention of this paper to impugn these findings. On the contrary in my own ethnomedical field research, I also encountered strong resistance to condom use in Rwanda. However, by merely reporting these statistics without attempting to make sense of them according to Rwandan standards of meaning, the authors allow readers to interpret the findings according to their own presuppositions. This opens the door to the possibility that readers of the article might conclude that Rwandans are an obdurate, irrational lot, impervious to the lessons of Western science. What I wish to demonstrate in this paper is that resistance to condom use makes perfect sense once we understand something about the way the person is socially constructed in Rwanda. Moreover, I feel that a 'mechanical model' of personhood, whose outlines I will sketch in this paper, can be usefully wedded to the 'statistical model' employed by the above authors and that this will enhance our understanding of sexual practices in Rwanda and potentially benefit health planners, for in order to devise culturally appropriate methods of dealing with AIDS in Rwanda, we need to take implicit cultural constructs seriously.

Before looking at the nature of Rwandan personhood, however, let us consider what it implies to employ a statistical model in a problem of this nature. Statistical studies of behaviour are built upon the assumption that aggregate or group behaviour can be summated from any number of more or less disparate individual behaviours. This approach is basically transactional. It presumes that society is equal to the sum of its parts and contractually engendered by the aggregate effect of different individuals leading their separate lives and choosing from a multitude of options. Epistemologically speaking, this assumption tends to introduce a fundamental division between the individual and society. While this dichotomy may be useful in some instances, in others it may lead us to ignore that many social phenomena are synergistic; they are more than the sum of their parts. Such phenomena cannot be fully understood merely by focusing one's attention on the associated behavioural components. Instead, we should view these aspects of social practice holistically, in the words of the sociologist Marcel Mauss as 'total social phenomena'.

Mauss's prime example of a 'total social phenomenon' is the concept of the 'gift'. The 'gift' is nothing if not synergistic; insight into it cannot be gained by simply summating different individual acts of giving and receiving. As a meaning, the 'gift' transcends separate instances of its occurrence in social life, and its implications permeate what are commonly thought to be distinct social institutions (of a religious, legal, moral, or economic nature). Using a variety of ethnographic examples, Mauss demonstrates that the ideology of the 'gift' encompasses the individual in his various exchange behaviours, while it also serves as a fundamental source of social meaning. The 'gift' implies the self, but a self whose behaviour cannot be abstracted from that of a relational other, another to whom the self is bound in reciprocity. As I will demonstrate in this paper, Mauss's insights can be usefully applied to the Rwandan notion of the 'gift'. These insights can help us to understand something about Rwandan attitudes towards the use of condoms.

Statistical and mechanical models
The distinction between transactional and holistic approaches corresponds in part to that between statistical and mechanical models. Statistical models employ explanatory elements that are different in scale from the phenomena which they represent. Mechanical models, on the other hand, use explanatory elements that are of the same scale as the phenomena which they represent. While sociology tends to employ statistical models generated from studies of large numbers of individuals, socio-cultural anthropology tends to concentrate on small population samples and to generate mechanical models in explanation. Neither model is inherently superior. Depending upon the level of explanation, either type of model may be more appropriate. Questions regarding the encompassing logic or rationale constitute the domain of the 'mechanical model'. For here the task involves unearthing principles which operate more or less independently of personal choice. At this level, it is not useful to envision the individual as a countable monad ontologically separate from society. It is not useful to envision the individual apart from society, for the group implies itself in the individual and conversely, the individual exists as a social being to the extent that he participates in the same universe of meanings as his fellows. The individual and society are mutually implicating, relational entities. The group constructs the individuals that comprise it and is constructed in its turn. The person is neither singular nor plural. He is perennially incomplete, ever involved in the process of being added to, built upon, and produced by the gifts of others. Through his own gifts, the person is habitually adding to and producing others. At any moment in this process, he is a 'fractal person,' a notion borrowed from the mathematical concept of fractality: 'a dimensionality that cannot be expressed in whole numbers'.

In contrast to our Western representation of discrete individuality where the isolated person is taken for granted as the analytically apposite unit at the basis of social action, in many non-Western societies, it is still too early to speak of individualism in quite the same way. The Western notion of the person posits both singularity and plurality. The individual is singular and the group is plural. We see the whole in terms of its parts and we infer the quality of the whole by merely adding up the parts. This corresponds to our notions of social action and it colours our perception of risk. Risk itself becomes a question of singularity and plurality, a question of chance and probability. Actuarial science devotes itself to computing risk in this way, though one should emphasize that its 'science' is based upon assumptions concerning the nature of the person that are peculiar to our culture.

In medical matters this tendency translates itself in the following way, 'What are one's chances of contracting disease X, if one adopts behaviour A, what are one's chances of contracting the disease, if one adopts behaviour B, etc.' Our depiction of medical risk almost always reflects this numbers game involving singularity and plurality. Representing risk in this manner and our penchant to see it as cross-culturally valid, has a lot to do with our positing of social relations in terms of singular individuals operating in consonance or dissonance with a plural collective.

Although many people in Rwanda are quite Westernized and doubtlessly somewhat influenced by the mode of thought I have just sketched, the fact that there appears to be general rejection of condom use would indicate that risk there is perceived differently. In my opinion, the Rwandan conception of risk is filtered through the eyes of a 'fractal person'. This person perceives his social universe not in terms of monadic individuals, but in terms of holistic structures of meaning whose patterns repeat themselves in slightly varying forms like the contours of a fractal topography, and whose implications reverberate through the apparently distinct social domains of exchange, sexuality, and health.

I maintain that 'fractality' is expressed primarily through the media of liquids and their passage from one body to another or their passage through the human body. These liquids include bodily secretions such as blood, semen, maternal milk, vaginal secretions, and saliva; liquids involved in social exchange such as cow's milk, sorghum beer, sorghum porridge, banana wine, and honey; and finally the primary fluid of terrestrial fertility, rainfall.

Pre-colonial representations of the 'fractal person'
In pre-colonial Rwandan society the most exemplary 'fractal being' was the king. Producing the king's body depended upon the gifts (or tribute) he received from others. But conversely, the physical well-being of everyone in the kingdom was dependent upon the prosperity thought to emanate from the king. The king's person was perceived as directly implicated in the fertility processes of land, cattle, and human beings. When fertility failed, as in drought, epizootic, or epidemic, the king could be executed or deposed.

The king's person was frequently depicted in myth, in both a figurative and a literal way, as a catalyst to promote the movement of fertility fluids. For example, the Rwandan supreme being, termed *Imaana*, was thought to be a 'diffuse, fecundating fluid' of celestial origin. The king embodied *imaana*, while his body served as the primary conduit through which this celestial beneficence passed in its descent from sky to earth, to all of Rwandan humanity. Thinking in analogical terms, the king's body resembled a hollow tube, open at the top and at the bottom. There is strong evidence that Rwandans themselves thought of the king's body in this way. The king, acting through ritual, was the foremost rainmaker for the entire polity and the owner of all Rwandan cattle whose ultimate origin had been the sky. It was said that the king drank the milk milked by the Creator, *Imaana*, while ordinary humanity drank the milk milked by the king.

The king's diet consisted almost uniquely of the prestigious liquid aliments of milk and beer. His body was produced then, from the quality of fluidity. Quite logically, anything which might compromise the movement of fluids in the king's body was thought to be inauspicious. We see this in the custom whereby the king was given a powerful purgative every morning. The king's mode of ingestion and his mode of excretion thus tended to follow the principle of fluidity or 'flow'.

If Rwandan well-being as a polity was dependent upon the movement of fluids, pathology in a collective sense arose either where this process was 'blocked,' or where it was allowed to proceed uncontrollably. More frequently, it was the imagery of 'blockage' that received attention. Drought was more feared than inundation, although separate royal rituals existed to counter either situation. 'Blockage' in the female body was an especially 'marked' condition. Girls of child-bearing age who had not developed breasts (perceived as lacking the capacity to produce milk) or who had never menstruated (perceived as lacking the capacity to produce blood) were the nemesis of the king. Their bodily state of 'blockage' could bring about drought or vitiate the fertility of the land in other ways. It was the king's responsibility to see that in both cases, such girls were put to death or banished.

The point of these examples is to demonstrate the interpenetration of notions about the person and notions about collective well-being. Both are elaborated in relation to one another and both are based on analogies which depict individual physiological processes as causally related to collective prosperity and fertility. According to this cosmology, it does not make sense to consider the individual as a singularity, i.e. a countable unit. Risk in this scheme of things would have to be conceptualised not in terms of probabilities, but in terms of the contagion of 'blockage'. In pre-colonial Rwanda, if an adolescent girl's body were 'blocked,' or if the king's body were 'blocked,' this quality could be transmitted to the entire collective and destroy it. Therefore, when one thought of danger and risk in pre-colonial Rwanda, one thought of the condition of 'blockage'.

Rwandan notions of the person today
Although Rwanda has undergone considerable transformation since the time that the first Catholic mission was established in 1900, a Rwandan way of living the body has tended to persist. This is manifest in the domain of consumption. A decided emphasis upon the ingestion of liquid aliments, for example, continues to characterize social occasions ranging from ordinary hospitality to celebrations of rites of passage. Rwandan drinks lend themselves to the expression of reciprocity and sociability, for they must be distributed and consumed within a relatively short time. Social relations are thus affirmed and reinforced in virtually all acts of drinking which involve alcoholic beverages or milk. When Rwandans visit one another, they

almost always offer their guests something to drink. Beverages of choice include manufactured beer, sorghum beer, banana beer, milk, and sorghum porridge. Furthermore, the beverages exchanged between visitors and guests are thought to contribute to the bodily constitution of the person receiving the liquid gift. On ordinary occasions, this is implicit in the exchange: on ceremonial occasions this is somewhat more explicit. When a woman gives birth, for example, she observes a period of seclusion. The termination of this period is socially demarcated by a visit to the household from friends and relatives of the couple. Many of the visitors bring gifts to the new mother. The wife's parents recompense their daughter in a special way. They bring her and her husband cow's milk, beer, a goat, and especially an important quantity of sorghum porridge, a liquid food which is supposed to encourage the new mother's lactation. The idea behind this custom, I believe, is that if the woman drinks sorghum porridge in sufficient quantity, she will have abundant maternal milk with which to breastfeed her child.

The wife's parents, therefore, will have aided their daughter's lactation through this gift of porridge and they will have indirectly participated in the production of the child's body through their gift. This custom manifests the cooperation which should obtain between agnatic and uterine kin in assuring the baby's development.

The end of the mother's seclusion period is also the moment when the newborn child is brought out and shown to other members of the family and immediate community. But this rite of passage can only be performed after the child's body has been examined and found to be free of anal malformations. People at this occasion receive a meal, especially the children present who are given favourite foods. These children in turn bestow a nickname on the newborn. The meal given to the children is termed 'to eat the baby's excrement,' for it is sometimes said that a small quantity of the baby's faecal matter is mixed with the food. This appellation may seem ironic, but in reality it celebrates the fact that the baby's body, in similar fashion to the body of the king in former days, has been found to be an open conduit, an adequate vessel for perpetuating the process of 'flow'. In a sense, the baby's faeces are its first gift and the members of his age class are its first recipients. The children at the ceremony incorporate the child into their social group by symbolically ingesting one of his bodily products. Their bestowal of a name upon the infant manifests their acceptance and reciprocity of his gift.

The image of the baby's body as an 'open' conduit is a socio-moral image as much as it is a physiological one. If the baby's body were 'closed' at the anal end, the baby would still be able to ingest, though not to excrete. The baby would be able to receive, but unable to give up or pass on that which it had received. In effect, its body would be a 'blocked' conduit. In social terms, such a body would be unable to participate in a reciprocity network, for while it could receive, it could never give. The construction of the moral person in Rwandan society then, is contingent upon two separate but related processes: first, it is contingent upon the exchange of gifts between kin. Secondly, the construction of the moral person is contingent upon the social attestation that the person correctly embodies the physiological attributes which analogically evoke the capacity to reciprocate, i.e. the capacity to perpetuate the process of 'flow'. The very term for 'man' in Kinyarwanda, *umugabo*, incorporates this ideal, for it is derived from the verb *kugaba* which means 'to give'.

The notion of the gift defies characterization merely in terms of singular individuals and plural groups. The 'gift' situates us in the social imagery of reciprocity, in the realm of 'fractal' beings. Such beings are ever-involved in the process of compensating the incompleteness or 'fractality' of others by adding to them with their gifts. In no other realm of Rwandan social experience is the idea of uncompleteness of 'fractality' more appropriate than in sexuality and reproduction. In Rwanda, ideas related to sexuality and human fertility are encompassed by ideas related to the 'gift' and to reciprocity. The term *intanga*, for example, which designates either the male or female potentiality to produce new life, means 'gift of self'. New life is produced when male *intanga*, or 'gift of self,' which are contained within a man's semen, fuse with female *intanga*, which are contained within a woman's blood. According to Rwandans, the most propitious moment for this to occur is during the first week following menstruation and after the couple have both had orgasm in coitus.

Rwandan sexual practices emphasize the reciprocal flow of secretions between the two partners, and demonstrate the importance Rwandans attach to female sexual response. In the Rwandan mode of intercourse, the man externally stimulates the woman's clitoris by tapping his penis against it. It is only after the woman has begun to experience orgasm and to produce copious vaginal secretions, that he penetrates her. The Kinyarwanda term for this kind of sex is 'to make urinate'. The man is supposed to make the woman urinate, i.e. cause her profuse vaginal secretion, before he himself ejaculates. Once again, therefore, sex follows the mode of 'flow/blockage' imagery and the ideal of reciprocity. Both partners procure pleasure from one another, while their two 'gifts of self' fuse to produce a common product, a child. One act of coitus, however, is not thought to be sufficient to bring about conception. On the contrary, conception is said to be a process which is dependent upon the continued admixture of male semen with female blood.

Placing a condom between the two partners, therefore, means interposing 'blockage' between the reciprocal flow of their secretions. It means turning male semen back upon itself. As we have seen from the other examples of 'flow/blockage' imagery in Rwandan culture, it also involves the danger or the risk of contagion. A woman risks becoming a 'blocked being' when her partner wears a condom. Hence the fear, widespread among women, that the condom would remain lodged in the vagina after intercourse. This also explains the reasoning behind some of the other most frequently raised objections against the use of condoms. For example: (1) the possibility of diminished pleasure. Because the reciprocal movement of fluids is emphasized in Rwandan lovemaking, it is difficult for Rwandan women to imagine how this could still occur while a condom is being used. (2) The possibility that disease might result from their usage or that condoms are unsafe. Because pathology according to Rwandan schemes of meaning has always been conceived in terms of 'flow' and 'blockage,' it is difficult for Rwandan women to imagine that a 'blocking' device could also be a healthful device. Less frequently cited reasons including: mistrust of one's partner and the fear of diminished fertility, can also be explained by this model. Wearing a condom, i.e. interposing an obstacle between oneself and one's partner, hardly expresses trust. Furthermore, as we have seen from pre-colonial Rwandan examples, 'blockage' was once associated with infertility.

Conclusion

While statistical studies often point to empirically valid aspects of behaviour and to risky behaviours, they sometimes ignore the rationale which gives rise to these behaviours. This tendency is particularly apparent in cultures where risk is not perceived in terms of quantities. In the Rwandan case, risk is perceived in terms of holistic schemes of meaning which penetrate seemingly disparate cultural realms and which reflect the indigenous concept of the person. In Rwanda the person is never socially constructed according to notions of discrete quantity; the person is neither a singularity as an individual, nor a plurality as a group. Instead, a more useful way of looking at the person in Rwanda involves the notion of fractality. The notion of fractality helps us to see Rwandan personhood as a dynamic process where people are constantly producing each other through their gifts. This core notion receives expression through the movement of fluid substances, substances which participate directly in terrestrial and human productivity, but yet are also important symbols in mythical discourse, in rites of passage, in everyday acts of exchange, and in sexuality.

In order to fully understand sexual practices and risk in Rwanda, therefore, one must look beyond numbers to the meaning of sex within the overall constellation of Rwandan values regarding social life and personhood. While statistical models are useful; there is a strong tendency in Western medical science to overestimate their importance. Medical researchers are prone to mistrust qualitative argument and to insist upon numbers as the final arbiter of truth, the so-called 'bottom line'. This has something to do with our tendency to see social relations in Western society in terms of quantitative images, a tendency which is implicit in concepts like 'maximization,' images which reflect our way of envisioning social relations in our society. Despite the fact that Rwandans are beginning to internalise Western cognitive constructs as they become progressively more absorbed into the global economy, the perspective of Western commodity culture will only take you so far in Rwanda. Then one has to look at the person beyond the number.

↻ Feedback

1 'Fractal person' is used to designate a Rwandan notion of personhood that emphasizes continuities between persons instead of stressing the person's boundaries, and appreciates inter-personal flows as affirming and life-giving. The term is borrowed from mathematics to describe, how 'holistic structures of meaning whose patterns repeat themselves in slightly varying forms' giving shape to very different dimensions of social life, including the sexual domain. In this view of personhood, bodily intercourse is an event of confluence, from which not only spring children, but from which also the health and wellbeing, the body and the person are (re)created.

2 If one conceives of sex in its modern Western sense, as aiming for personal, individual satisfaction, in which confluence plays a minor role, a condom may be a nuisance, but it does not touch upon the ultimate purpose of sex. If one, however, regards substantial confluence as constitutive of personhood, a condom hits the core of bodily intercourse.

3 Taylor himself makes the following recommendations:

While the above model of Rwandan cultural constructs might seem to preclude the immediate adoption of condom use, I believe that Rwandans will eventually accept them as an effective measure against the propagation of AIDS. In a public relations campaign aimed at educating Rwandans to the AIDS implications of various sexual practices, one should begin by working in consonance with the above cultural constructs rather than at counter current to them. While some unmarried Rwandan women have chosen abstinence as a way of avoiding AIDS, short of abstinence, the practice of kunyaza (the specifically Rwandan form of wet vaginal sexual intercourse) should be encouraged. Well-lubricated vaginal walls probably offer some degree of protection against the propagation of AIDS. Furthermore, female prostitutes and the Rwandan males who frequent them – who show higher rates of HIV seropositivity – are less likely to practice kunyaza. In this instance the male's concern is for his own pleasure and not for that of his partner, while the female prostitute's principal concern is monetary. Thus added to the fact that female prostitutes increase their risk of contracting HIV infection by virtue of their greater number and variety of sexual contacts, it is also likely that they are more frequently obligated to engage in relatively dry vaginal intercourse. As a step toward non-penetrative intercourse, kunyaza could also be promoted. Since penetration is delayed until relatively late in the sexual act with kunyaza, it might be suggested to Rwandan males that they dispense with penetration altogether during non-procreative sex. Furthermore, kunyaza could be extolled as a half-way measure toward the use of a condom. Because kunyaza entails a great deal of external clitoral contact, the wearing of a condom would not interfere with this aim. Health planners could encourage Rwandans to practice their culturally specific form of intercourse but with the added element of using a condom. This would constitute building upon an already existing and traditionally valued practice rather than attempting to introduce something which might otherwise seem entirely new, unfamiliar, and opposed to Rwandan cultural constructs. (Taylor 1990: 1027–8)

Body, person and power

The previous section discussed the consequences of a particular notion of person-hood for bodily practice and health. The question arises whether personhood in its embodied form simply determines behaviour, like a cultural programme, or whether it could also be challenged, altered or mixed. This section will look at instances, in which culturally shaped notions of embodied personhood, through people's bodies, engage with and renegotiate social order. Personhood emerges here not only as the imprint of society on the person, but also as a resource with which people can shape their place in society. The body is both a site towards which the expectations of one's society and culture are applied, and the place from which the person engages with other people, and with culture and society. It is both structured and structuring, acting and acted upon.

An example of such enmeshing of cultural ideas and bodily practice is possession by spirits or ancestors, which can be found almost everywhere in the world. In modern European society, possession has over the past two centuries been progres-sively converted into mental illness. Thus, the possession of women was, during the nineteenth century, reconceptualized as hysteria, which was attributed to migratory movements of the womb in the female body. This implied that the origin of the afflicted women's behaviour was no longer sought in their social relations but inside their bodies. Thus individualized and medicalized, hysteria was transformed further into the conceptual language of psychiatry, and the treatment of the possessed (or the hysterical) changed, often replacing broader social engagement with confinement and medical treatments that 'experts' applied to women's bodies.

Today, possession remains an accepted interpretation of particular female behaviours in parts of rural southern and south-eastern Europe, including Turkey, and outside Europe it often remains a dominant idiom of dealing with certain forms of female affliction. Here, possession may be seen as beneficial or empowering (as in shamanic possession), as a threat (as in demonic possession) or as sickness. It can be at once scary, debilitating and empowering, as may be found in the biographies of healers and diviners in various parts of East Africa: they are first possessed and fall ill, then they are treated by healers who bring the possessing spirits under control, and eventually they become healers themselves, making fruitful use of the capacities of their spirits. Below, we will first look at the example of a socially well-accepted spirit possession cult, and then at a situation in which possession engages with oppression and medicalization in a conflict about culture and labour.

Possession and the 'overdetermined person'

In anthropology, possession has often been read as an expression of social tension between the possessed and her surroundings. According to an older thesis, possession was used as a covert individual strategy to achieve one's end in social conflicts, for example by women to extract resources from their dominant husbands (Lewis 1970). More recent approaches studied possession as an aspect of 'resistance' to repressive societal orders, such as the old South African regime (Comaroff 1985). While the first approach retains an emphasis on the person's mind governing and using her body, the latter focuses more on the body itself. Far from being a mere thing upon which other people (including the owner) exercise power, the body is seen as an active participant, engaging in relations with others and with their expectations and power. The body is where it happens: the inscription of power, the conflicts and the resistance.

The anthropologist Janice Boddy has explored these issues suggestively, looking at the example of Sudanese women who are taken up into the Zar cult, a ritual community of possessed women (1988). Boddy shows how Sudanese women's personhood is conceptualized as 'closed': moral values associated to femininity contrast closedness, equalling moral good, to openness, equalling moral badness. This personhood, which is elaborated in moral tales and everyday conversations, is inscribed onto the female body by, among other practices, circumcision and infibulation (closing the body). Women's daily practices and the objects they engage with enforce this ideal of closedness, creating an enduring habitus: their bodies are shaped by these social values, and their bodies, thus transformed, shape their social actions. These ideas about gender and gendered bodies, and openness and closedness, are pervasive in Sudanese society, but women are the ones who, through their bodies, have to bear the weight of it. Boddy calls this the 'overdetermination of the women's selfhood'.

With the term 'overdetermined', Boddy draws attention to the fact that the cultural image of person and body as closed is contradicted by the expectation of female fertility:

> . . . the closed moral self-image women are enjoined to assume, cannot always be sustained by experience. In this lies an ambiguity inherent to morality – between what is and what ought to be – which their continuous socialization may eventually fail to overcome: the woman who is, by definition, 'morally appropriate fertility' may experience infertility or some other significant contravention of her feminine self-image. (Boddy 1988)

Possession by Islamic spirits, *djinn*, which makes the women go into trance and act as men, Europeans and other radically different kinds of person, tends to occur at junctures in the women's lives when embodied habitus and expectations of fertility collide.

Possession, often preceded by sickness, radically opens these closed women's selves, inverting the rules of closedness and subverting gendered moralities. In possession, the woman becomes another person than the one she is or should be: an outsider, open, amoral. She can act out conflicts around the closed personhood (and bodies) she usually lives in: 'through possession, women can step outside their everyday world and gain perspective on their lives'. Whether this can bring about improvements and changes to her life remains an open question. One could argue that it creates the opportunity for dialogue and change, but as an institutional mechanism of debate it also contributes to maintain a shared body of experiences and values. However, the membership in the Zar cult that results from the treatment of possession and gives the affected women a social grouping of their own, implies an achievement of status and a source of support.

Body, spirit and resistance

Boddy chooses to analyse female possession as part of a non-Western, Muslim and African culture. The following text by Aihwa Ong looks instead at possession in a modern, capitalist context. Female factory workers from a cultural background that endorses spirit possession, become possessed at work. Here, one question is why women get possessed in the factory – and in this way the article takes up Boddy's argument. Another question is, how different groups construct possession. This, in turn, casts light on the relationship between how the body and person are constructed by possession, and how they are understood by biomedicine in the context of capitalist production. Possession is not just an event that stands up against or within certain power relations, but it can also be an object of power, shaped and reframed by political, scientific and economic power. Here the body is not only a locus of domination and resistance, but also of the reinterpretation of such resistance. Possession becomes a mental illness calling for biomedical attention, and the resistant commentary is lost.

Activity 10.2

Read the abridged article by Ong (1988) below with the following questions in mind:

1   Why, according to the Malay concepts of social order, would young women in factories be visited by spirits?
2   How does the biomedical categorization of the women's deviant behaviour as 'mental illness' and its treatment with tranquillizers support the women's continuous exploitation?
3   Discuss Ong's alternative, anthropological categorization of the women's behaviour as a 'complex negotiation of reality'.

The production of possession: spirits and the multinational corporation in Malaysia

The sanitized environments maintained by multinational corporations in Malaysian 'free trade zones' are not immune to sudden spirit attacks on young female workers. Ordinarily quiescent, Malay factory women who are seized by vengeful spirits explode into demonic screaming and rage on the shop floor.

Management responses to such unnerving episodes include isolating the possessed workers, pumping them with Valium, and sending them home. Yet a Singapore doctor notes that 'a local medicine man can do more good than tranquillizers'. This paper will explore how the reconstitution of illness, bodies, and consciousness is involved in the deployment of healing practices in multinational factories.

Anthropologists studying spirit possession phenomena have generally linked them to culturally specific forms of conflict management that disguise and yet resolve social tensions within indigenous societies. In contrast, policymakers and professionals see spirit possession episodes as an intrusion of archaic beliefs into the modern setting. These views will be evaluated in the light of spirit possession incidents and the reactions of factory managers and policymakers in Malaysia. I believe that the most appropriate way to deal with spirit visitations in multinational factories is to consider them as part of a 'complex negotiation of reality' by an emergent female industrial workforce. Hailing from peasant villages, these workers can be viewed as neophytes in a double sense: as young female adults and as members of a nascent proletariat.

Furthermore, their spirit idiom will be contrasted with the biomedical model to reveal alternative constructions of illness and of social reality in the corporate world. I will then consider the implications of the scientific medical model that converts workers into patients, and the consequences this therapeutic approach holds for mending the souls of the afflicted.

Economic development and a medical monologue on madness
As recently as the 1960s, most Malays in Peninsular Malaysia lived in villages, engaged in cash cropping or fishing. From the early 1970s onward, agricultural and industrialization programs induced the large-scale influx of young rural Malay men and women to enter urban schools and manufacturing plants set up by multinational corporations. Throughout the 1970s, free-trade zones were established to encourage investments by Japanese, American, and European corporations for setting up plants for offshore production. In seeking to cut costs further, these corporations sought young, unmarried women as a source of cheap and easily controlled labour.

Before the current wave of industrial employment for young single women, spirit possession was mainly manifested by married women, given the particular stresses of being wives, mothers, widows, and divorcees. With urbanization and industrialization, spirit possession became overnight the affliction of young, unmarried women placed in modern organizations. The dismissal of Malay interpretation of spirit events by Western-trained professionals became routine with the large-scale participation of Malays in capitalist industries. A 1978 paper entitled 'How to Handle Hysterical Factory Workers' complained that 'this psychological aberration interrupts production, and can create hazards due to inattention to machinery and careless behaviour'. The author classified 'mass hysteria' incidents according to 'frightened' and 'seizure' categories, and recommended that incidents of either type should be handled 'like an epidemic disease of bacteriological origin'. The biomedical approach called for the use of sedatives, 'isolation' of 'infectious' cases, 'immunization' of those susceptible to the 'disease,' and keeping the public informed about the measures taken. This and other papers on spirit possession episodes in modern organizations adopt the assumptions of medical science which describe illnesses independent of their local meanings and values. 'Mass hysteria' is attributed to the personal failings of the afflicted, and native explanations are denigrated as 'superstitious beliefs' from a worldview out of keeping with the modern setting and pace of social change. 'A monologue of reason about madness' in the philosopher Michel Foucault's terms was thereby introduced into Malaysian society, coinciding with a shift of focus from the afflicted to their chaotic effects on modern institutions. We will need to recover the Malays' worldview in order to understand their responses to social situations produced by industrialization.

Spirit beliefs and women in Malay culture

Spirit beliefs in rural Malay society are part of the indigenous worldview woven from strands of animistic cosmology and Javanese, Hindu and Muslim cultures. Since the 1960s, the widespread introduction of Western medical practices and an intensified revitalization of Islam have made spirit beliefs publicly inadmissible. Nevertheless, spirit beliefs and practices are still very much in evidence. Invisible beings unbounded by human rules, spirits come to represent transgressions of moral boundaries, which are socially defined in the concentric spaces of homestead, village, and jungle. This scheme roughly coincides with Malay concepts of emotional proximity and distance, and the related dimensions of reduced moral responsibility as one moves from the interior space of household, to the intermediate zone of relatives, and on to the external world of strangers.

The two main classes of spirits recognized by Malays reflect this interior-exterior social/spatial divide: spirits associated with human beings, and the 'free' disembodied forms. It is free spirits that are responsible for attacking people who unknowingly step out of the Malay social order. Free spirits are usually associated with special objects or sites marking the boundary between human and natural spaces. These include (a) the burial grounds of aboriginal and animal spirits, (b) strangely shaped rocks, hills, or trees associated with highly revered ancestral figures, and (c) animals like were-tigers. As the gatekeepers of social boundaries, spirits guard against human transgressions into amoral spaces.

From Islam, Malays have inherited the belief that men are more endowed with reason than women, who are overly influenced by human lust. Their spiritual frailty, polluting bodies, and erotic nature make them especially likely to transgress moral space, and therefore permeable by spirits. Although men are also vulnerable to spirit attacks, women's spiritual, bodily, and social selves are especially offensive to sacred spaces, which they trespass at the risk of inviting spirit attacks. In everyday life, village women are bound by customs regarding bodily comportment and spatial movements, which operate to keep them within the Malay social order. When they blur the bodily boundaries through the careless disposal of bodily exuviae and effluvia, they put themselves in an ambiguous situation, becoming most vulnerable to spirit penetration.

Until recently, unmarried daughters, most hedged in by village conventions, seem to have been well protected from spirit attack. Nubile girls take special care over the disposal of their cut nails, fallen hair, and menstrual rags, since such materials may fall into ill-wishers' hands and be used for black magic. Menstrual blood is considered dirty and polluting, and the substance most likely to offend spirits. This concern over bodily boundaries is linked to notions about the vulnerable identity and status of young unmarried women. When young Malay women break with village traditions, they may come under increased spirit attacks as well as experience an intensified social and bodily vigilance.

Since the early 1970s, when young peasant women began to leave the village and enter the unknown worlds of urban boarding schools and foreign factories, the incidence of spirit possession seems to have become more common among them than among married women. I maintain that like other cultural forms, spirit possession incidents may acquire new meanings and speak to new experiences in changing arenas of social relations and boundary definitions. In village society, spirit attacks on married women seem to be associated with their containment in prescribed domestic roles, whereas in modern organizations, spirit victims are young, unmarried women engaged in hitherto alien and male activities. This transition from village to urban-industrial contexts has cast village girls into an intermediate status that they find unsettling and fraught with danger to themselves and to Malay culture.

Spirit visitations in modern factories
In the 1970s, newspaper reports on the sudden spate of 'mass hysteria' among young Malay women in schools and factories interpreted the causes in terms of 'superstitious beliefs,' 'examination tension,' 'the stresses of urban living,' and less frequently, 'mounting pressures' which induced 'worries' among female operators in multinational factories. Multinational factories based in free-trade zones were the favoured sites of spirit visitations. Reports of such incidents reveal that spirit possession, believed to be caused by defilement, held the victims in a grip of rage against factory supervisors. Furthermore, the disruptions caused by spirit incidents seem a form of retaliation against the factory supervisors. In what follows, I will draw upon my field research to discuss the complex issues involved in possession imagery and management discourse on spirit incidents in certain Japanese-owned factories.

The cryptic language of possession
Young, unmarried women in Malay society are expected to be shy, obedient, and deferential, to be observed and not heard. In spirit possession episodes, they speak in

other voices that refuse to be silenced. Since the afflicted claim amnesia once they have recovered, we are presented with the task of deciphering covert messages embedded in possession incidents.

Spirit visitations in modern factories with sizable numbers of young Malay female workers engender devil images, which dramatically reveal the contradictions between Malay and scientific ways of apprehending the human condition. What is being negotiated in possession incidents and their aftermath are complex issues dealing with the violation of different moral boundaries, of which gender oppression is but one dimension. What seems clear is that spirit possession provides a traditional way of rebelling against authority without punishment, since victims are not blamed for their predicament. However, the imagery of spirit possession in modern settings is a rebellion against transgressions of indigenous boundaries governing proper human relations and moral justice.

For Malays, the places occupied by evil spirits are nonhuman territories like swamps, jungles, and bodies of water. These domains were kept distant from women's bodies by ideological and physical spatial regulations. The construction of modern buildings, often without regard for Malay concern about moral space, displaces spirits, which take-up residence in the toilet tank. Thus, most village women express a horror of the Western-style toilet, which they would avoid if they could. Besides their fear of spirits residing in the water tank, an unaccustomed body posture is required to use the toilet. In their hurry to depart, unflushed toilets and soiled sanitary napkins, thrown helter-skelter, offend spirits who may attack them.

A few days after the spirit attacks in an American factory, I interviewed some of the workers. Without prompting, factory women pointed out that the production floor and canteen areas were 'very clean' but factory toilets were 'filthy'. A spirit haunted the toilet, and workers, in their haste to leave, dropped their soiled pads anywhere. A worker remembered that a piercing scream from one corner of the shop floor was quickly followed by cries from other benches as women fought against spirits trying to possess them. The incidents had been sparked by spirit visions, sometimes headless, gesticulating angrily at the operators. Even after the spirit healer (*bomoh*) had been sent for, workers had to be accompanied to the toilet by foremen for fear of being attacked by spirits in the stalls.

My fieldwork elicited similar imagery from the workers in two Japanese factories based in the local free-trade zone. In their drive for attaining high production targets, foremen were very zealous in enforcing regulations that confined workers to the work bench. Operators had to ask for permission to go to the toilet, and were sometimes questioned intrusively about their 'female problems.' Menstruation was seen by management as deserving no consideration. Foremen sometimes followed workers to the locker room, terrorizing them with their spying. One operator became possessed after screaming that she saw a 'hairy leg' when she went to the toilet. A worker from another factory reported: Workers saw 'things' appear when they went to the toilet. Once, when a woman entered the toilet she saw a tall figure licking sanitary napkins. It had a long tongue, and those sanitary pads cannot be used any more. This lurid imagery speaks of the women's loss of control over their bodies as well as their lack of control over social relations in the factory. Furthermore, the image of body alienation also reveals intense guilt (and repressed desire), and the felt need to be on guard against violation by the male management staff who, in the form of fearsome predators, may suddenly materialize anywhere in the factory.

As mentioned above, spirit attacks also occurred when women were at the work bench, usually during the 'graveyard' shift. A factory operator described one incident: 'It was the afternoon shift, at about nine o'clock. All was quiet. Suddenly, the victim started sobbing, laughed and then shrieked. She flailed at the machine . . . she was violent, she fought as the foreman and technician pulled her away. She did not know what had happened . . . she saw a were-tiger. Only she saw it, and she started screaming. People say that the workplace is haunted by the spirit who dwells below . . . Well, this used to be all jungle, it was a burial ground before the factory was built. The devil disturbs those who have a weak constitution.' Spirit possession episodes then were triggered by black apparitions, which materialized in 'liminal' spaces such as toilets, the locker room and the prayer room, places where workers sought refuge from harsh work discipline. Other workers pointed to the effect of the steady hum and the factory pollutants, which permanently disturbed graveyard spirits. Unleashed, these vengeful beings were seen to threaten women for transgressing into the zone between the human and nonhuman world, as well as modern spaces formerly the domain of men. By intruding into hitherto forbidden spaces, Malay women workers experienced anxieties about inviting punishment.

In Malay culture, it is incumbent upon young women to conduct themselves with circumspection and to diffuse sexual tension. However, the modern factory is an arena constituted by a sexual division of labour and constant male surveillance of nubile women in a close, daily context. The shop floor culture was also charged with the dangers of sexual harassment by male management staff as part of workaday relations. To combat spirit attacks, the Malay factory women felt a greater need for spiritual vigilance in the factory surroundings. The fear of spirit possession thus created self-regulation on the part of workers, thereby contributing to the intensification of corporate and self-control on the shop floor. Thus, as factory workers, Malay women became alienated not only from the products of their labour but also experienced new forms of psychic alienation. Their intrusion into economic spaces outside the home and village was experienced as moral disorder, symbolized by filth and dangerous sexuality. Some workers called for increased 'discipline,' others for Islamic classes on factory premises to regulate interactions between male and female workers. Thus, spirit imagery gave symbolic configuration to the workers' fear and protest over social conditions in the factories. However, these inchoate signs of moral and social chaos were routinely recast by management into an idiom of sickness.

The worker as patient
Taylorist forms of work discipline are taken to an extreme in the computer-chip manufacturing industries set up by multinational corporations in Malaysia. However, I would argue that the recoding of the human body-work relation is a critical and contested dimension of daily conduct in the modern factory. Struggles over the meanings of health are part of workers' social critique of work discipline, and of managers' attempts to extend control over the work force. The management use of workers as 'instruments of labour' is paralleled by another set of ideologies, which regards women's bodies as the site of control where gender politics, health, and educational practices intersect.

In the Japanese factories based in Malaysia, management ideology constructs the female body in terms of its biological functionality for, and its anarchic disruption of, production. These ideologies operate to fix women workers in subordinate positions in systems of domination that proliferate in high-tech industries. A Malaysian investment brochure advertises 'the oriental girl,' for example, as 'qualified by nature and inheritance to contribute to the efficiency of a bench assembly production line'.

Within international capitalism, this notion of women's bodies renders them analogous to the status of the computer chips they make. Computer chips, like 'oriental girls,' are identical. For multinational corporations, women are units of much cheap labour power repackaged under the 'nimble fingers' label.

The abstract mode of scientific discourse also separates 'normal' from 'abnormal' workers, that is, those who do not perform according to factory requirements. In the factory environment, 'spirit attacks' was often used interchangeably with 'mass hysteria'. In the managers' view, 'hysteria' was a symptom of physical adjustment as the women workers 'move from home idleness to factory discipline.' This explanation also found favour with some members of the work force. Scientific terms like 'hysteria sickness', and physiological preconditions formulated by the management, became more acceptable to some workers.

In corporate discourse, physical 'facts' that contributed to spirit possession were isolated, while psychological notions were used as explanation and as a technique of manipulation. In another factory, a *bomoh* was hired to produce the illusion of exorcism, lulling the workers into a false sense of security. The personnel manager claimed that unlike managers in other Japanese firms who operated on the 'basis of feelings,' his 'psychological approach' helped to prevent recurrent spirit visitations. Regular *bomoh* visits and their photographic images were different ways of defining a social reality, which simultaneously acknowledged and manipulated the workers' fear of spirits.

Medical personnel were also involved in the narrow definition of the causes of spirit incidents on the shop floor. A factory nurse periodically toured the shop floor to offer coffee to tired or drowsy workers. Workers had to work eight-hour shifts six days a week and allowed little time for workers to recover from their exhaustion between shifts. The shifts also worked against the human, and especially, female cycle; many freshly recruited workers regularly missed their sleep, meals, and menstrual cycles. Thus, although management pointed to physiological problems as causing spirit attacks, they seldom acknowledged deeper scientific evidence of health hazards in microchip assembly plants. Through psychological readings, the causes of spirit attacks produced in the factories were displaced onto workers and their families.

In corporate discourse, both the biomedical and psychological interpretations of spirit possession defined the affliction as an attribute of individuals rather than stemming from the general social situation. Scientific concepts, pharmaceutical treatment, and behavioural intervention all identified and separated recalcitrant workers from 'normal' ones; disruptive workers became patients. In one factory, the playing out of this logic provided the rationale for dismissing workers who had had two previous experiences of spirit attacks, on the grounds of 'security.' This policy drew protests from village elders, for whom spirits in the factory were the cause of their daughters' insecurity. The manager agreed verbally with them, but pointed out that these 'hysterical, mental types' might hurt themselves when they flailed against the machines, risking electrocution. By appearing to agree with native theory, the management reinterpreted spirit possession as a symbol of flawed character and culture. The sick role was reconceptualised as internally produced by outmoded thought and behaviour not adequately adjusted to the demands of factory discipline. The worker-patient could have no claim on management sympathy but would have to bear responsibility for her own cultural deficiency. The non-recognition of social obligations to workers lies at the centre of differences in worldview between Malay workers and the foreign management. By treating the signs and symptoms of disease as 'things-in-themselves,' the biomedical model freed managers from any moral debt owed the workers. Afflicted and 'normal' workers alike were made to see that spirit possession was nothing but confusion and delusion, which should be abandoned in a rational worldview.

The work of culture: hygiene and dispossession
Modern factories transplanted to the Third World are involved in the work of producing exchange as well as symbolic values. Medicine, as a branch of cosmopolitan science, has attained a place in schemes for effecting desired social change in indigenous cultures. While native statements about bizarre events are rejected as irrational, the conceptions of positivist science acquire a quasi-religious flavour. In the process, the native 'work of culture,' which transforms motives and affects into 'publicly accepted sets of meanings and symbols,' is being undermined by an authoritative discourse that suppresses lived experiences apprehended through the worldview of indigenous peoples.

To what extent can the spirit healer's work of culture convert the rage and distress of possessed women in Malaysia into socially shared meanings? As discussed above, the spirit imagery speaks of danger and violation as young Malay women intrude into hitherto forbidden spirit or male domains. Their participation as an industrial force is subconsciously perceived by themselves and their families as a threat to the ordering of Malay culture. Second, their employment as production workers places them directly in the control of male strangers who monitor their every move. These social relations, brought about in the process of industrial capitalism, are experienced as a moral disorder in which workers are alienated from their bodies, the products of their work, and their own culture. The spirit idiom is therefore a language of protest against these changing social circumstances.

Luddite actions such as breaking machines in a state of possession in stalling production reverse momentarily the arrangement whereby work regimentation controls the human body. However, the workers' resistance is not limited to the technical problem of work organization, but addresses the violation of moral codes.

Spirit possession episodes may be taken as expressions both of fear and of resistance against the multiple violations of moral boundaries in the modern factory. They are acts of rebellion, symbolizing what cannot be spoken directly, calling for a renegotiation of obligations between the management and workers. However, technocrats have turned a deaf ear to such protests, to this moral indictment of their woeful cultural judgments about the dispossessed. By choosing to view possession episodes narrowly as sickness caused by physiological and psychological maladjustment, the management also manipulates the *bomoh* to serve the interests of the factory rather than express the needs of the workers. Spirit possession incidents in factories made visible the conflicted women who did not fit the corporate image of 'normal' workers. By standing apart from the workaday routine, possessed workers inadvertently exposed themselves to the cold ministrations of modern medicine, rather than the increased social support they sought. Other workers, terrified of being attacked and by the threat of expulsion, kept up a watchful vigilance. This induced self-regulation was reinforced by the scientific gaze of supervisors and nurses, which further enervated the recalcitrant and frustrated those who resisted.

Spirit possession episodes in different societies have been labelled 'mass psychogenic illness' or 'epidemic hysteria' in psychological discourse. Different altered states of consciousness, which variously spring from indigenous understanding of social situations, are reinterpreted in cosmopolitan terms considered universally applicable. In multinational factories located overseas, this ethnotherapeutic model is widely applied and made to seem objective and rational. However, we have seen that such scientific knowledge and practices can display a definite prejudice against the people they are intended to restore to well-being in particular cultural contexts. The reinterpretation of spirit possession may therefore be seen as a shift of locus of patriarchal authority from the *bomoh*, sanctioned by indigenous religious beliefs, toward professionals sanctioned by scientific training.

In Third World contexts, cosmopolitan medical concepts and drugs often have an anaesthetising effect, which erases the authentic experiences of the sick. More frequently, the proliferation of positivist scientific meanings also produces a fragmentation of the body, a shattering of social obligations, and a separation of individuals from their own culture. In Malaysia, medicine has become part of hegemonic discourse, constructing a 'modern' outlook by clearing away the nightmarish visions of Malay workers. However, as a technique of both concealment and control, it operates in a more sinister way than native beliefs in demons. Malay factory women may gradually become dispossessed of spirits and their own culture, but they remain profoundly dis-eased in the 'brave new workplace'.

↻ Feedback

1 Malay culture precisely defines relations between the generations and genders and emphasizes regulated transitions in a person's life course. The factory setting puts young women in situations, for example vis-à-vis their supervisors, that make the maintenance of these norms impossible. Possession arises in the tension between the values of personhood outside the factory and the demands on the person selling her labour within the factory.

2 Biomedicine, as practised within these factories, accepts the given order of work and social relations as rational. Possession, which disturbs the production, is defined as irrational, or mental illness. It is thus given a place within the rationality of the factory, and the critical potential of the women's experience is devalued. The possessed women become 'dis-possessed' of their culture but remain 'dis-eased' in the workplace.

3 Categorizing spirit possession as a 'complex negotiation of reality' implies an appropriateness of the women's behaviour as response to, and debate about, specific, inhumane conditions. If one, by contrast, thinks that these conditions have to be accepted, if only for the time being, as the reality of offshore industrial work within globalized capitalism, possession is a mental illness that misrepresents the given reality and requires treatment. Yet, even if one does not accept the inhumane workplace and the conditions of exploitation, one might argue that the women will only actively change these if they organize collectively in labour unions, whereas possession, as an individualized response, fails to wield political power.

Summary

In this chapter we have introduced different notions of personhood – such as individuality and 'dividuality' or 'fractality' – that are variously emphasized in different societies and at different times. Personhood and morality are not primarily intellectual issues located in peoples' minds, but part of bodily life and experience. This makes them natural to those who embody them, and as a result they change less rapidly than, say, verbal, formal knowledge. We explored, moreover, how the body can be employed to challenge dominant notions of personhood and to resist power that is brought to bear upon it. Thus, we saw how an overdetermined mode of female personhood is inscribed upon the body, enacted and reaffirmed by bodily practice, and potentially challenged and renegotiated through specific bodily actions. Moreover, we saw the role of sickness in the renegotiation of repressed personhood and as embodied resistance to exploitative and oppressive regimes. Finally, we noted the role that biomedical discourses can play in subduing and normalizing such resistance.

References

Boddy J (1988) Spirits and selves in northern Sudan: the cultural therapeutics of possession and trance. *American Ethnologist* 15: 4–27.

Bourdieu P (1977) *Outline of a Theory of Practice*. Cambridge: Cambridge University Press.

Comaroff J (1985) *Body of Power, Spirit of Resistance*. Chicago: Chicago University Press.

Geissler PW (1998) 'Worms are our life.' Understandings of worms and the body among the Luo of western Kenya (parts 1 and 2). *Anthropology and Medicine* 5: 63–81 and 133–44.

Geissler PW, Prince RJ. Persons and relations in Luo plant medicine. In: Plants, health and healing. Explorations on the interface of medical anthropology and ethnobotany. Hsu E & Harris S (eds) 2005. Oxford: Berghalin Publishers.

Hoskins J (1998) *Biographical Objects. How Things Tell the Stories of People's Lives*. New York: Routledge.

Lewis IM (1970) A structural approach to witchcraft and spirit possession, in Douglas M (ed) *Witchcraft Confessions and Accusations*. London: Tavistock.

Ong A (1988) The production of possession: spirits and the multinational corporation in Malaysia. *American Ethnologist* 15: 28–41.

Parkin D (1995) Latticed knowledge. Eradication and dispersal of the unpalatable in Islam, medicine, and anthropological theory, in Fardon R (ed) *Counterworks. Managing the Diversity of Knowledge*. London and New York: Routledge.

Schumaker L (in press) *The Madness of Poverty and the Medicine of Complaint: Music, Healing and Struggle in Twentieth-Century Zambia*.

Strathern M (1988) *The Gender of the Gift. Problems with Women and Problems with Society in Melanesia.* Berkeley: University of California Press.

Taylor CC (1990) Condoms and cosmology: the 'fractal' person and sexual risk in Rwanda. *Social Science and Medicine* 31: 1023–8.

Taylor CC (1992) *Milk, Honey and Money. Changing Concepts in Rwandan Healing.* Washington: Smithsonian Institution Press.

Medical research

11

Overview

This chapter emphasizes the importance of medical research for perceptions of and responses to biomedicine and public health in economically deprived societies. Medical research projects and other health interventions are not conducted upon an empty slate, but in a context that has grown over time and accumulated multiple layers of historical experience that can be accessed through people's memories. In Africa, these are to a large extent memories of colonial occupation and the exploitation and oppression that went with it. In this chapter, we explore the weight of this past for present health research and intervention.

Learning objectives

By the end of this chapter you should:

- **recognize the influence of colonial and postcolonial history for the implementation of contemporary medical research and medical intervention**
- **understand some of the potential unintended implications of medical research in African societies**

Key terms

Colonial occupation The formal, politically and militarily supported, domination and control of territories inhabited by people with another identity, language or culture and a different political constitution, who have not explicitly consented to occupation with the intent of transforming their societies, cultures, and the aim of benefiting economically (and otherwise) from this.

Discipline Adapted from the late philosopher Michel Foucault to designate modern forms of social order that apply power to bodies in non-coercive ways. An example of a 'regime of bodily discipline' would be the colonial emphasis on 'hygiene', which transformed domestic and interpersonal practices, reorganized public and private space, and instilled an order of cleanliness and separations that not only reduced disease but also transported concepts of the person, relations and morality that were part of colonial governance (Fabian 1991: 159–61).

Postcolonial A qualification of periods, societies, nations or ideas after formal colonial occupation; sometimes used as impartial temporal definition but more commonly to draw attention to the lasting impact of the colonial period.

The context of medical field research

The academic, political and economic context of medical field research in Africa has changed in the course of the past century, but the basic social constellation has remained similar: groups of highly trained and mobile experts (from local and overseas research institutions) with large resources and wide-ranging networks, together with locally recruited and trained field staff, conduct investigations among less well-endowed and educated, relatively locally stable, mostly rural study populations. These social relationships – marked by hierarchical differences in knowledge, wealth and power – and the social networks that are formed as part of research among different scientists and within African populations, are usually seen by medical researchers as mere background to the 'real' task of scientific discovery. This background is considered irrelevant unless problems in this social context jeopardize the scientific data collection or the quality of the data.

From an anthropological perspective, by contrast these social relations are an essential part of the scientific and medical endeavour. They produce different knowledges: that of laypeople about biomedicine, and that of scientists about local people, including scientists' knowledge about local people's health. Medical scientists often assume that the only significant aspect of fieldwork is numeric data collection, and the only significant proportion of knowledge consists in the scientific results that eventually translate into health policy, but the anthropological view is that everything that happens in or around a medical research project and every idea that is generated by the encounter between researchers and researched is significant for the overall effects of medical research. For example, the order and procedures of specimen collection should not be regarded as a mere means towards an end, but as a social constellation that reflects, negotiates and constitutes social relations (see Figure 11.1). Analysing such relations, studies of the social effects of health research could be instructive for the planning of larger, sustainable health interventions based upon this research. We will return to this understanding of medical research as an open network of social relations.

Before we continue, a comment on the place of medical research in relation to the health system. In Western industrialized society research is, from the patients' point of view, a peripheral domain compared to the therapeutic role that doctors and hospitals play. By contrast, in sub-Saharan Africa and other economically deprived areas, research offers vital services – such as treatment and prevention of disease – which are otherwise often unavailable for ordinary citizens. The misconception that research is a mere complement to existing health services leads to an underrating of its potential power in such settings. Moreover, since the beginning of colonial occupation, medical research has often provided the first contact that people had with biomedical practice. As a result, it has left an imprint on people's ideas about biomedicine and their relations with medical institutions. Because of its history and its disproportionate importance within contemporary health provision, medical research provides us with an excellent topic to investigate the logic and practice of biomedically grounded health interventions.

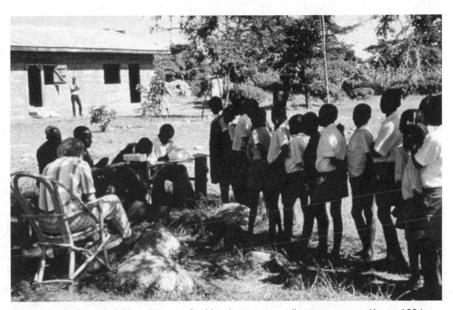

Figure 11.1 School children lining up for blood-specimen collection, western Kenya, 1994 (photograph Wenzel Geissler)

Medicine and colonialism

In discussions about the impact of colonial occupation on African peoples, medicine remained for a long time the one firmly positive contribution as it had undoubtedly saved lives. Some held that medicine had only saved relatively few lives among the colonized but had been used tactically to convince Africans of, for example, the power of Christianity; others countered that, especially during early colonial occupation, medicine had been too weak to convince the colonized people – although it did convince the colonizers of their own benevolence. Others again argued that medical discourses fed into racial segregation and supported imperialism. More recently medicine has come under scrutiny by historians and anthropologists looking not just at what good medicine does in medical terms but at what it did on the whole to Africans and colonial and post-colonial social relations (for example, Vaughan 1991).

Some authors argued that biomedicine and colonialism 'are cut from the same cultural cloth' (Comaroff and Comaroff 1993), implying that their relationship is not a matter of the former serving as a tool of imperialism but that the two sets of knowledge and practice have emerged interdependently. The constitution of Africa as a continent to be discovered, conquered and dominated went along with ideas of Africa as a sick continent in need of cure, and with the scientific quest for new diseases and treatments in African bodies. The constitution of modern African persons and colonial subjects was shaped both by political and economic forms of domination and governance and by the introduction of new bodily regimes, and in turn, resistance to and renegotiation of colonial governance took place around bodily practices, healing and medical ideas.

This historical association between biomedicine and imperialism is relevant for public health. If biomedicine and public health have been shaped by the interrelation between medical concerns and political and economic governance in colonial times, and if fundamental aspects of colonial relations continue to define the place of African societies in the world, then it is necessary to reflect on how the relationships between medicine, health, politics and economy are articulated in particular contexts in order to understand the working of public health and develop interventions.

Colonial medical research

In this section we will look more closely at the history of tropical medical research. Sub-Saharan Africa was formally occupied by European nations for almost three generations (roughly from the 1880s to the 1960s). While some parts of Africa had experienced European power and economy earlier through the transatlantic slave trade, this direct occupation introduced novel political and economic structures, and new knowledges, such as Western medicine and Christianity. After formal independence the overt political aspects of the occupation disappeared but there were continuities throughout this period, and some problems have even been exacerbated. Even where important changes in ideas, attitudes and actions did occur, the traces of the past continue to exercise their influence on the present through memories. This applies to large political-economic structures such as land ownership as much as to specific institutions and practices, such as medical research, and often both dimensions of the past intersect.

Sleeping sickness research was a medical activity that combined scientific investigations and public health interventions, and was deployed and developed almost continuously throughout colonial and postcolonial times, transforming people's bodies and the landscapes they lived in, and leaving mixed memories. In East Africa, it began with the Ugandan Medical Officer (MO 1898–1906) ADP Hodges' expeditions along the shores of Lake Victoria. His diaries give some idea of these modest beginnings.

19.1.1902 'Got note that I am to go to K. to investigate the "sleeping sickness" which has become prevalent here.' This involves 2–3 months travel by canoe along the lake and into the hinterland.

5.2.1902 'First cases of sleeping sickness.' Hodges is actively searching cases and taking blood samples. He treats other illnesses he encounters until he runs out of drugs.

20.2.1902 'In L. District. The taking of blood for examination, the poor souls look upon as a cure apparently, akin to vaccine. I say nothing about it. I daren't undeceive them or they would not come at all. I wish I had something to give them. I give arsenic, they simply rush for it and crowd for it.'

9.3.1902 Emissaries from one of the islands come with a delegation to Hodges and present him with sheep, asking him to come to treat sleeping sickness. Hodges declines and takes the delegation's blood. They force him to accept sheep to thank him and he promises to visit them later.

9.3.1902 Hodges mentions that there is a famine and that he lacks food for the 30 men with whom he travels along the lakeshore.

23.3.1902 Canoeing along the shore, Hodges observes more and more sickness and abandoned villages, which he attributes to sleeping sickness.

26.5.1902 Back in his HQ in Jinja, Hodges invites a medicine man who says he can cure sleeping sickness to work alongside him in his dispensary.

'I have seen 22 of his cases. They aren't, I think, cured, but all profess to be much better and some are certainly so. I am going to let him try on some of my cases to test his medicine, which is the root of a tree, which is common here. I hope, but I am in no way convinced that there is anything in it.'

7.6.1902 The mentioned medicine man comes to the hospital. He treats with baths and ointments made from a tree and bleedings from scalp and legs. Hodges comments: 'The scarification of the scalp is not unscientific and relieves the headache generally.'

18.6.1902 Later, however, he concludes: 'The native cure seems of doubtful success, at any rate for the time.'

(Rhodes House Archives, MSS.Afr.s.1782)

Hodges is at this point of his career a scientist in a lonely and thus careful position, maintaining positive relations with the local people, who are surprisingly eager to provide blood samples. Hodges depends upon the studied peoples, not only for specimens, but also for food and shelter; he is still a visitor rather than an occupant. The diary shows respect and curiosity towards indigenous knowledge. While later public health interventions often relied upon a stark dichotomy between scientific ideas and local 'superstitions', Hodges, like other doctors working in Africa earlier in the nineteenth century (Livingstone, for example) does not yet find himself in a position to distinguish his own 'knowledge' from others' 'beliefs', but shows genuine interest in the local healer, whose knowledge eventually turns out to be just as inconclusive as Hodges' own ideas. However, there are also misunderstandings, as the study populations believe that bleeding treats them, and Hodges refrains from confronting them with the truth, fearing to lose his specimens.

Sleeping sickness research and control continued in the same area up to the 1960s. As colonial occupation became more efficient, it began to transform people's lives and livelihood. Campaigns involved sometimes forced collection of blood specimen. If people were diagnosed positive they were taken to treatment camps at a distance from their homes, where they were given month-long treatments, which were feared because of their sometimes lethal side effects. Some infested areas were cleared of their inhabitants, who were resettled elsewhere, and only after decades was the land opened up for resettlement (often causing lasting conflicts). In many endemic areas, the landscape was systematically transformed by new, unfamiliar patterns. During the first epidemic, Hodges himself devised geometrically shaped clearings designed to separate tsetse flies, cattle and humans (see Figure 11.2; Hoppe 1997); in later campaigns, bush clearing, the building of access roads and insecticide spraying of the lakeshore were critical to disease control, and created lasting memorials of research and disease control in the landscape (see the discussion of modernist interventions in Chapter 1).

These activities provided people with contradictory experiences. On the one hand, the potent treatment of a deadly disease demonstrated biomedicine's abilities. The

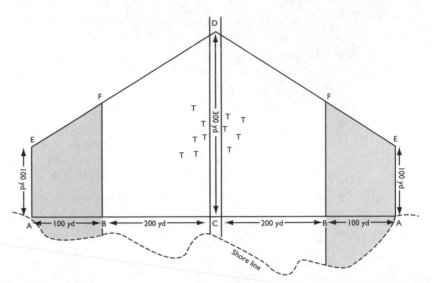

Figure 11.2 Hodges' clearing diagram. C-D travel route, B-F-D-C area cleared, B-C-B cleared shore with access allowed, A-E-F-B areas cleared but access prohibited. (Based on drawing in Hodges, 1911:6, from Hoppe 1997)

long-term control of sleeping sickness conveyed a sense of the technical power of the government. On the other hand, however, the often painful measures that were employed also gave this power an ambivalent dimension. Moreover, in as much as successful disease control demonstrated power, the neglect of sleeping sickness control in recent decades and the return of tsetse flies reveals the weakness or carelessness of later governments. Thus, negative and positive memories and their links to negative and positive experiences in the present provide the ground for different, potentially contradictory, reactions to contemporary research and health interventions.

The ambiguity is captured in the story told about the origins of sleeping sickness, that inhabitants of one of the Kenyan sleeping sickness areas told in 2000:

> During the early colonial years, when the leading local clan was at war with other local clans (a conflict that had been triggered by colonial allocations of political power), one of the factions sent for powerful medicine to a medicine-man in Uganda where the epidemic originated, triggered by colonial mobility. The messengers returned with an earthen pot, which contained the eggs of tsetse flies. The pot was hidden in the bush, where an ignorant farmer smashed it and released the plague, which depopulated the land people had fought over.

This narrative of the foreign origin of epidemic and its political links to colonialism and colonial mobility is still told today. Here, an outside power creates local conflicts and is drawn upon to exacerbate these to the effect of generalized destruction. This story is not just an explanation of how sleeping sickness, a previously unknown scourge, came about, but also a reflection of people's recognition that it arrived at the same time as colonial occupation. The narrative links the experience of sickness and death to social decay and disintegration. The source of death and disintegration is located outside the community, whence it is brought inside through the collaboration of a local group.

This narrative resembles stories, told in the same area today, about the origins of HIV/AIDS. This scourge (distinguished from sleeping sickness as 'the death of today' as opposed to 'the death of long ago') emerged into public consciousness in the late 1980s, a period of political violence between government and opposition. Western Kenya, the opposition stronghold, was also most heavily affected by HIV/AIDS. When people discussed the origins of AIDS in the early 1990s, they linked ethnic, political, geostrategical and medical concerns in rumours, which accused the government, supported by the United States of America (Kenya's Cold War ally), of spreading HIV through donated condoms in order to eliminate the people of western Kenya and the opposition (which at some point had expressed socialist leanings). As in the case of sleeping sickness, ill health, health interventions and politics on various levels merged into one explanatory narrative.

Narratives like these continue to shape responses to public health interventions in the area. For example, the rumours about the American origin of HIV/AIDS, linked to politics and racism, have provoked negative responses to condom promotion, HIV awareness campaigns and research projects. People are keenly aware of the different origins of research projects and donor initiatives, and respond more suspiciously to those from some nations than to others.

Thus, the memories and stories people tell about a century of medical research and intervention are alive in contemporary African societies, and they are evoked to make sense of and respond to present-day interventions. Medical anthropologists in public health have the task of revealing and examining these memories in particular populations and areas and helping to take them into account in the planning and implementation of health work.

Imaginations of research

While medical science created an imagination of 'the diseased heart of Africa', many of the occupied peoples produced equally striking imaginations of colonial medicine. One of these was the idea that Europeans, and in particular white medical doctors, took people's blood (or body parts) in order to sell them, thus killing or sterilizing Africans. These narratives were first documented in the Congo in the early years of the last century (Ceyssens 1975), and spread, possibly with connections to India and the Arab world (Pels 1992), throughout central, eastern and southern Africa, where they were occasionally described by colonial administrators or researchers. Thus one of the fathers of medical anthropology, Evans-Pritchard, noted, in the 1930s: 'There is some humour to be found in the fact that many Azande (Southern Sudan) were convinced that the British doctors were cannibals, and performed operations to obtain meat to satisfy this disgusting propensity' (Evans-Pritchard 1960: 257).

While most commentators found these stories amusing or attributed them to 'African tradition' or 'superstition', others related them to the experience of colonial occupation and its exploitative and oppressive aspects, and interpreted them as 'resistance' to the colonial regime. Others again have analysed them more closely as historical sources in their own right, expressing specific and varied colonial experiences in locally meaningful idioms (White 2000).

✏️ **Activity 11.1**

Look at the *White Lions* depicted by the Zairian painter Tshibumba as part of a series of pictures about the colonial experience, and answer the following questions.

1 What are the main features of colonial body-snatching emerging in Tshibumba's painting, and what do they signify?
2 What would you argue, from an anthropological point of view, if somebody said that these narratives were expressions of 'superstition' or 'traditional belief'?
3 Why, do you think, were medical researchers, game rangers and gold prospectors frequently implicated in these rumours?

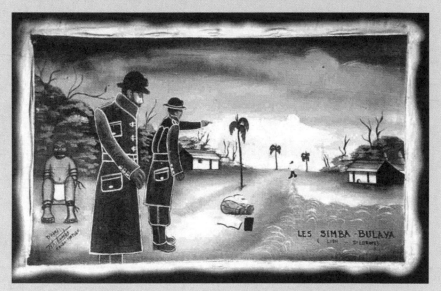

Figure 11.3 'White Lions' (from Fabian 1996)

↻ **Feedback**

1 The main features of the painting are:
   • the White Lions operate along the road – they come from outside and enter the community to find their victims
   • they arrest unsuspecting victims in the village, picking them at random
   • the victims are tied and gagged, powerless, ready to be slaughtered
   • one of the perpetrators has white skin, the other one, who seems to act, has black skin – reflecting colonial hierarchy and collaboration
   • both wear uniforms that might resemble laboratory (or medical) coats, combined with miners' helmets – representing possibly a variety of colonial experiences (medicine, mines, fire brigades – White 2000)

- both 'lions' wear protective glasses and gloves and their bodies are covered almost completely, in contrast to the undressed victim – emphasizing the power differential between them and the refusal of direct bodily contact by the evil intruders, who make use of the victims' bodies.

These features embody dimensions of the colonial experience:

- mobility: intrusions from outside
- anonymity and unrelatedness: 'lions' and 'locals' do not know each other, and the lions' uniforms and protective dress make them 'unknowable'; they explicitly refuse to enter social relations
- uniforms: linking medical, economic, military and other interventions in one uniformed framework
- collaboration: co-operation of some Africans with the occupants' regime.

2 These narratives reflect particular conditions and relations, and should not just be brushed away as superstition, but heard and understood. The concept of tradition implies some unspecified tie to an African past, whereas the blood-stealing narratives presented above are part of recent colonial experiences. Traditional ideas (such as witchcraft) that resemble blood-stealing accusations are dissimilar in that the former accuse local people from within the community of trying to magically harm their neighbours; in contrast, blood-stealing agents do not care about their victims but use them to make a profit; they prefer people they have no relation to, unlike witches who normally strike at their neighbours and kin.

3 Answers to this question depend upon local context. A common trait of researchers, prospectors and rangers is that they behave conspicuously: they follow people, guard wild animals, or criss-cross the bush to dig holes; they do not follow a recognizable social pathway (for example, visiting people) but move in trajectories that from a local perspective are hard to place in a meaningful pattern; they have unknown resources at their disposal, and, more importantly, they take away things and find great value in substances that from a local perspective are worthless (such as wild animals, which they don't eat, earth, blood and faeces (= stool). This makes them remarkable; and a satisfied and confident population might just have poked fun at them; but people under duress or with anxieties about their livelihood and health react negatively to them or attribute their predicament to them.

Summary

This chapter showed that medical research projects and other health interventions are not conducted in a vacuum, but in a context that has developed over time and accumulated multiple layers of historical experience that can be accessed through people's memories. In Africa these are, to a large extent, memories of colonial occupation and the exploitation and oppression that went with it. These negative experiences, and the many positive experiences that some Africans have had with biomedicine, with research, and even with colonial occupation, are not always expressed as a straightforward political or economic critique, but take often the shape of stories and rumours, such as those about blood stealing. Such narratives warrant further study in the social context within which they are told and used to achieve particular ends.

References

Ceyssens R (1975) Mutumbula: mythe d'opprimé. *Culture et Development* 7: 483–550.

Comaroff J and Comaroff J (1993) The diseased heart of Africa. Medicine, colonialism, and the black body, in Lindenbaum S and Lock M (eds) *Knowledge, Power, and Practice: The Anthropology of Medicine and Everyday Life*. Berkeley: University of California Press.

Evans-Pritchard E (1960) Zande cannibalism. *Journal of the Royal Anthropological Institute* 90: 257.

Fabian J (1991) Religious and secular colonization, in *Time and the Work of Anthropology. Critical Essays 1971–1991*. London: Harwood Academic Publishers.

Fabian J and Tshibumba KM (1996) *Remembering the Present. Painting and Popular History in Zaire*. Berkeley: University of California Press.

Hoppe KA (1997) Lords of the fly: colonial visions and revisions of African sleeping sickness environments on Lake Victoria 1906–1961. *Africa* 67: 86–106.

Pels P (1992) Mumiani: the white vampire. A neo-diffusionist analysis of rumour. *Etnofoor* 5: 165–87.

Vaughan M (1991) *Curing Their Ills. Colonial Power and African Illness*. Cambridge: Polity Press.

White L (2000) *Speaking with Vampires: Rumor and History in Colonial Africa*. Berkeley: University of California Press.

12

Health interventions as a field of social practice

Overview

In this chapter we conceptualize the 'social network' of medical research – the trial community – as a field of ethnographic study. We discuss science as a 'social network' – as an activity that does not merely reveal truth or nature, but constitutes it in the context of concrete practices that connect different people and objects in dynamic networks. This involves not only studying the target populations of medical research and their responses to research, but also the medical researchers themselves, their practices, their funders and the policy makers behind them.

We show that in order to understand scientific knowledge and the knowledge and rumours that study populations produce about research, we must study these networks from an ethnographic perspective. We argue that medical anthropology can improve research and health intervention by revealing and exploring the wider networks of both intentional, unintended and unrecognized connections in which research is embedded.

Learning objectives

By the end of this chapter, you should have:

- broadened the anthropological focus from the conventional 'field' of localized communities to broader, translocal networks
- understood the nature of rumours as tools to deal with uncertainty in the context of medical research, and as instruments in local power struggles

Key terms

Debates An emphasis on debates in ethnographic fieldwork – in contrast to an emphasis on, for example, homogeneous local knowledge – takes into account the fact that no social group is homogeneous and that it is especially from open debates and confrontations that we can learn about local ideas and practices. Thus we ought to study not 'ideas of' social groups, but 'debates within' them.

Network Networks are different from social groups. They are potentially open ended, not defined by boundaries or a core, and can be extended and changed continuously. The term emphasizes the connections between different nodes, and the possibility of multiple connections of each node, rather than the essential identity of entities, such as a social group or the individual member of the group. What counts, is what links actors, not what they are by themselves.

Occult Used to designate explanations of social practice that refer to secret or unheard-of forces; the term 'magic' would earlier have been used, but this is now avoided because it connotes stereotypes such as that of African witchcraft. The concept allows the exploration of similarities between occult ideas in, for example, the United States (such as the idea that extraterrestrial aliens have assumed power in the White House) and in Africa (such as rumours about blood-selling politicians). It perpetuates the notion of fundamentally different knowledges – magical or occult, and scientific or rational – and cannot be a valid analytical term, but is instead a temporary label for an interesting field of anthropological inquiry.

Rumour Narratives, often orally distributed, that serve as a means to discuss experiences, reaching beyond the facts that are generally agreed on about these experiences, or combining known features in innovative ways. The power of rumours to make people act lies in the fact that they are not bound to agreed facts – one can believe in them and doubt them at the same time, and they can be neither proven nor falsified. Therefore, they can suddenly gain mobilizing force in a particular situation, and equally quickly dissolve and vanish from public debate and become 'just a story' again.

(Social) constructivism This approach to knowledge denies the existence of reality prior to human engagement and the validity of truth in the sense of a corresponding representation of reality. Instead, it poses that reality is whatever is known and that all knowledge is socially produced. Constructivism can thus lead to relativism as it allows no distinction between true and untrue statements.

Science as a social network

There are few anthropological studies of medical field research in resource-poor settings like Africa. Sometimes anthropologists are brought into a trial to ensure community participation or to solve a conflict with a study population, but there is generally little interest in studying, ethnographically, the totality of a research endeavour. The few existing social studies of medical research in Africa usually look 'down', at the target populations and their responses to research (see, for example, Molyneux *et al.* 2004). While such research is very worthwhile for understanding and improving medical research practices, medical anthropologists should also look 'up and around' – that is at their colleagues and their practices, their funders and the policy makers behind them.

Anthropological research in Euro-American scientific laboratories can provide some inspiration (for example Latour 1999). Participating in everyday laboratory work, anthropologists used participant observation as earlier anthropologists had done among other 'tribes' and wrote ethnographies of the scientists' tribe. They showed how scientists' activities and interactions constitute scientific facts, and how instruments, objects and substances are not just tools, or the inert substrate on which discoveries were grown, but active participants that contribute to the making and unmaking of discoveries. In other words, new scientific connections and social relations ought to be studied as a single productive process. This is the approach taken in the ethnography of medical trial communities in developing countries as well. Here, however, the scientific laboratory includes local people, not only instruments. The objects and the public of science overlap in the study subjects of population-based health research in Africa. This offers new insights into the constitution of the public understanding of science, and the scientific understanding of the public. Moreover, studies of community-based scientific practice in Africa allow us to reinsert everyday life and wider networks of relatedness, which laboratory-based science studies often neglected, into the picture. For all members of a rural African trial community research is part of community life and vice versa – community life becomes part of the trial practices.

To study how medical science is made we could, for example, study the day-to-day social relations and practices of field research. Fieldworkers play a crucial role in this (Fairhead *et al.* 2004). They are usually invisible in medical publications, which only present the scientists, as authors, and reduce the study populations to figures and diagrams. Yet, fieldworkers provide evidence of the importance of social relations in the production of research and health interventions: recruited from local populations they interact daily with researchers and researched, mediating the spheres that scientific ideas of knowledge production separate: those of observer and observed. As such they provide a useful entry for ethnographic study. Thus, a study we conducted of a malaria vaccination trial in the Gambia focused on the role of fieldworkers, who in this particular study were stationed in rural communities for over one year. Through their interactions with villagers and scientists the fieldworkers found pragmatic solutions for social problems in the trial, such as those relating to the fair distribution of health care benefits. In other words, they made or unmade the field.

Other, even less recognized actors, such as drivers, cleaners and data entry clerks, make contributions to science work. Other actors again are acknowledged in the publication of research findings, such as the principal investigators and study populations, but we know little about their relationships and internal group dynamics, and how these affect the scientific process. Beyond the actors in the 'field', there are the wider realms of the scientific community, of the non-scientific public, of funders, donors and policy makers. All these are part of the trial community that makes scientific research.

Activity 12.1

The aim of this activity is to extend our field of vision to the network of the global 'trial community', and transcend the focus on the local study population as the topic of ethnographic study.

Look at Figure 12.1, a cartoon from a Kenyan newspaper, which depicts a public controversy, in 1995, about the intellectual property rights in HIV-vaccine research, which a joint Kenyan-UK research team had conducted among young women in a poor part of Nairobi.

1 List all the actors and groups, institutions and sites in the picture, or draw a network map of this trial community.
2 What are the potentially significant relationships between these actors and in which ways they are important?
3 Which methods could be used to investigate particular relations within this intervention network?

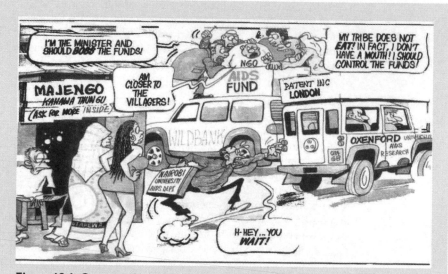

Figure 12.1 Cartoon published by the *East African Standard*, Kenya during the 1994–5 controversy about the patent rights regarding a potential HIV vaccine that had been tested by a collaborative research project between the University of Oxford and Kenya Medical Research Institute

Source: Paul Kelemba, *East African Standard*, Nairobi.

↻ Feedback

1 From left to right: the male clients of the prostitutes; their wives or neighbours; the prostitutes (study population); the Kenyan scientists; the Land Rover of the 'Oxenford' group; the UK scientists; the Land Cruiser of the World Bank and multilateral donors; the Kenyan AIDS community; politicians; Churches; NGOs.

2 Many could be suggested; among these are:

- scientists – study subjects (prostitutes) (the core of the trial)
- study subjects (prostitutes) – clients (the supposed background of the trial, but essential for its outcomes)
- Kenyan scientists – UK scientists (co-operation, competition; control of funds; control of results and publications)
- scientists – donors (competition for funding; politics and scientific aims; competing donors; policy and research)
- scientists – politicians (political interests; economic interests; national pride)
- global organizations – national organizations (postcolonial relations; domination; corruption; transnational elites)
- multilateral co-operation – cooperation with the ex-colonial occupier (see the Land Cruiser versus Land Rover distinction marking bilateral (UK) collaboration versus multilateral organizations) (memories; resentments; attitudes; shared experiences; knowledge of each other)

- and last not least: trial community (depicted here) – wider public (which reads the paper) (transparency; expectations; mistrust; national pride).

3 Possible methodological approaches (which should be combined) would include e.g.:

- ethnography of the scientists: living with and working with the scientists, for example, as an assistant, using participant observation
- interviews and group discussions in the political, NGO and donor sphere; possibly supplemented with participant observation in an NGO
- ethnography of the study population: residing in a slum area and learning about the daily life of the women, families and clients, and the context of the trial.

Rumours and debates about medical research

We now turn to the study community and to anxieties about research, not because most study populations have a negative attitude to health research but because these fears speak about the connections between medical research interventions and the life world of the study subjects, which more scientific views tend to relegate to the background. Study protocols and published papers focus on a single set of connections, set out by the study objectives – for example, the link between water contact and Bilharzia infection – but rumours and debates among the studied peoples link the scientists' actions to history and politics, to kinship and fertility, to economy and livelihood and even to religion. Rumours blur the sharp distinctions between what is relevant and what is not, and what is held together by established causal links and what is not, which scientists try to impose on a more messy reality. Because of their openness towards new connections, these debates can make us look afresh at medical research and health interventions.

Rumours like those about the white lions, often originating in colonial times, continue to circulate in Africa and are often applied to medical research projects. In recent years, anthropological interest in such narratives has grown, and they appear to have become more common under the impact of the confusion and violence of recent decades (see, for example, Comaroff and Comaroff 1999: 292). These rumours can be applied to a range of actors, but in Africa they often target medical research, although medical researchers mention them only rarely in their publications, as in this comment by Nchito et al. (2004) about a trial of iron supplementation in Zambia:

> Almost half the children . . . were not followed-up at 10-months. This huge loss to follow-up was partly due to respondent fatigue and partly to fears from rumours circulating in the country about blood thefts by so-called Satanists. The belief of the existence of a cult whose members drink human blood as part of their rituals, is quite widespread in Zambia . . . and has a long history . . . The collection of blood is generally viewed with much suspicion.

Although we could not find other examples in the literature, when we asked medical researchers with field experience in Africa, many of them contributed stories of similar rumours. Narratives about blood stealing or Satanism are found all over sub-Saharan Africa, and in much researched sites such as The Gambia accusations of blood selling are part of national mythology, known to both scientists and villagers (Fairhead *et al.* 2004). Such rumours make wide connections and travel far and fast. Thus in 2000, mothers in western Kenya learned from the national newspapers about a book linking HIV to early polio trials (Hooper 1999), and referred to this in their rejection of the ongoing polio vaccination campaign. Similarly, in 2003, study subjects in The Gambia knew about the 2002 Nigerian riots against polio vaccinations and related these to their own experiences with a malaria vaccine trial.

Most of these rumours are about bodies and body products, and often they emphasize blood, fertility, women and children. Research and health interventions, these narratives imply, are a threat to social relatedness, to the essence of life, and to its continuity. One way to analyse such rumours is to 'read' them as texts about the colonial experience (White 2000). This allows us to tease out hidden meanings, as one would do when interpreting a historical source. As social anthropologists, we are interested in what rumours can tell us about particular social relations within the network of a medical research project, and about how such relations change and develop in time.

Rumours can be employed to highlight problematic social ties on different levels. They often concern national politics and ethnicity, or even international economic and political relations. For example, Feldman-Savelsberg *et al.* (2000) showed how Cameroonian schoolgirls' fears about vaccinations expressed historical and political concerns that transcended the limited range of the vaccination campaign itself and linked gender, race and fertility, and politics and economy. Similarly, the widespread public suspicion of the combined measles, mumps and rubella vaccine (MMR) in Britain, which has continued for years despite considerable scientific evidence that the vaccine is safe, might be attributed to a wider sense of mistrust of the government and its health institutions that is particular to the social and political condition of the country as a whole.

Rumours are also entangled with smaller scale concerns, such as relations within a community, between neighbours and families. Rumours are made in face-to-face contacts, in talking, and used in local contexts. It is usually not the entire population that holds such views, but people discuss them and reach temporary consensus. Rumours are open-ended debates between people, rather than a fixed 'story'. Rumours are not stable, and whether people think they are important or not depends not just on the researchers or their project but at least as much upon the relations between people within the study community at a given moment in time.

For example, our project on the malaria vaccination trial in The Gambia studied a village that had collectively objected to a vaccine trial and had voiced suspicions about blood selling. In this village, one young man had an exceptionally high education from a prestigious scientific college but unfortunately no adequate employment due to the economic crisis. He had apparently been most vocal about the blood-selling allegations, and as one of the project fieldworkers put it: 'they listened to him, as he was a scientist himself'. Thus, despite his youth, even older people were ready to listen to him in this case, as he was formally trained, and evidently happy to underline his status in this way. Although his dress and comportment suggested a youthful, urban, possibly religiously inspired, anti-Western defiance, we cannot tell his precise motives for supporting the rumour. Whatever his motives, they vanished when he befriended the project fieldworker based in his village – a similarly bright, educated young man – and he even became a solid supporter of research leading his village into the trial. The case illustrates is that it is often individuals, their social ties and experiences and specific personal motives that make and unmake rumours, and not just historical memories or collective political experiences and that relations between villagers and between researchers and researched contribute to producing as well as transforming such stories.

Micro-level interactions and the macro-level explanations are not mutually exclusive, as people in a local setting enact global connections: the young man had studied science in a former colonial college and found no work partly due to reduced government spending, which in turn was related to overseas donor policies. He had lived abroad, had a broad worldview and experiences well beyond the local. Thus, rather than presenting purely local relations and conflicts, colonial and postcolonial tensions are reflected and transformed on the micro-level of social interaction.

The experience of one author (Geissler 2005), in 1994, as a student of medical parasitology in a western Kenyan village further illustrates such local processes of rumour. The category that people applied to him (locally referred to as *kachinja*), was similar to the white lions: white people with black assistants driving in white Land Rovers along the tarmac road and catching villagers to drain their blood. According to local informants, the narratives about *kachinju* were shaped by the colonial wars and colonial medical research, much as earlier readings of blood-stealing rumours had shown. But despite these similarities between the narratives throughout history and across eastern Africa, the local actions and relations it produced at this moment were specific to the given situation, when the researcher arrived in the village he called Uhero (Geissler 2005):

✎ Activity 12.2

Now read the following extract:

📖 The uses of *kachinja*

The following narratives show how the *kachinja* idiom is engaged in social relations and situations. The first case concerns a primary school teacher with whom I got acquainted during the first days of the research; here an initial impression of mutual understanding gave way to a realisation of distance. The other case is about a larger family homestead, in which initial miscomprehensions and suspicions turned into a lasting engagement with each other.

Mr Osunga's dilemma

A dynamic, young headmaster at one of the study schools befriended us during the early stages of the study and invited us to lunch in his home, a well-kept compound of concrete houses with high trees, characteristic for the mission-educated old local elites. He belonged to a dominant clan of the area, and his father had been an assistant chief. He found it appropriate to welcome the overseas visitors, both out of friendliness, to provide his children an educational experience and to confirm his family's status in the area. He attended community meetings and tried to convince people of our good intentions and of the 'development' that our project would bring.

He told me about a boy who suffered from chronic illness and introduced me to the child's father, the owner of the local store, a successful, but somewhat secretive and little liked man. The child had a swollen liver and I offered to take a blood slide to our laboratory. A week later, I returned with the (negative) results of the examinations and was met with unusual hostility by the boy's father, who refused the offer to take the boy to the district hospital. Startled, I looked for my acquaintance in the school, hoping to get an explanation. The headmaster met me politely but was less welcoming that he had been and declined knowledge of the boy's case. Our relationship subsequently declined and reached rock-bottom when he at a parent-teachers' meeting agitated against our team referring to the blood-collections.

During the following year, I gathered some elements of an explanation: my relationship with Mr Osunga, the son of the late colonial chief, who had hosted the sleeping-sickness research teams operating in the area in the 1970s, had revived the idiom of *kachinja*. The shopkeeper, whose child's blood specimen I had taken, was widely believed to entertain spirits, which he had brought with him from the coast, to support his business. Rumour had it that these had to be fed on human blood, which he procured from people he killed. His son's illness was attributed to his victim's revenge. When the headmaster brought his white visitor one evening to backroom of the little shop in order to take a blood specimen from the very sick child, observers combined memories of colonial times with present social tensions and suspicions and since all three protagonists were concerned with blood, this served as the red thread in the (not completely coherent) narrative that connected them with each other, with the past, and with the wider world. As a result, Mr Osunga had to publicly dissociate himself from the presumed masters or *kachinja*. Hence his open rudeness, very uncommon in Uhero, towards me and our group.

At the time, Mr Osunga's volte-face terminated our social contact, but when I met him a year later at a community meeting, the conflict and the accusations were forgotten, and he asked me for medical advice. For a moment we both had got entangled in the *kachinja* idiom, but as our work raised less and less anxieties in the village, *kachinja* had become useless for both Mr Osunga's critiques and for his self-defence.

This encounter between two educated, economically entrepreneurial men of the locality and a traveling researcher shows the variability of the *kachinja* idiom, its multivalence, and its changing impact on social relations. It can designate people from different geographical origins, educated, political figures and wealthy people. It plays on associations of knowledge and money, colonial history and local politics; and it can change function in the social process in which it is evoked. While this case confirms familiar patterns of modern 'occult' accusations, pitching elite men against local peasants, the second case is more complex, and I think more characteristic for the uses of rumours.

Mr Okoth's family

Our first visits to the home of Mr Okoth, his four wives, two mothers, 16 children and 7 grandchildren, were friendly but distant. Mr Okoth was a proud host but his wives were aware of the *kachinja* rumours and suspicious about the research. They fulfilled the duties of hospitality but asked my research assistant hostile questions. Repeated visits to the second of Mr Okoth's wives established a closer relationship. She voiced her concerns but was satisfied by our explanations. However, this emerging friendship provoked the animosity of her younger co-wives, who now raised *kachinja* accusations against both the second wife and us. These accusations also reflected long-standing tensions between the different women in the household. The second wife had lost most of her children and took care of those who survived on her own, while her youngest co-wife had many children and was better supported by the husband. These long-term tensions had at other occasions been articulated in terms of 'evil eye' and accusations of sorcery. Under the impact of our sudden appearance, they temporarily took the shape of *kachinja*.

Eventually, we succeeded in restoring our relationships with all the wives. These friendly interactions with the women, though, provoked the hostility of Mr Okoth. Rumours reached us that he now publicly accused us of stealing blood or in any case of being self-interested and untrustworthy. When we first had come to his home, we had been his prestigious visitors, not least because he himself had been a public health technician until his retirement and had, as we learned later, worked in the 1970s as a field assistant for the sleeping sickness campaign. Based on this experience, he practiced as an 'injectionist' treating other villagers against common illnesses. Our visits to his 'office' at the centre of the homestead had confirmed his reputation. But when we had established friendly relations with his wives his association with the outside visitors turned other villagers against him and revived memories of the days when the sleeping sickness researchers had had their camp in his home. Led by a neighbour, some older men accused Mr Okoth of being a *kachinja*, collaborating with us to steal the village children's blood.

The neighbour in question, Mr Odhiambo, had an outspoken suspicion regarding white people. He was an orthodox member of Legio Maria, a syncretistic Catholic church, and the only person I met in Uhero who occasionally wore a hide, which made some villagers suspect that he may have been a MauMau freedom fighter. As an immediate neighbour, he disagreed with Mr Okoth, who was Anglican, about religion, and he had old land conflicts with Mr Okoth's family, and his clan, which partly stemmed from the resettlement of the area after sleeping sickness. The thrust of Mr Odhiambo's accusations concerned Mr Okoth's former state employment and his work with research and blood-collection, which made him a likely *kachinja* working on behalf of remote power-holders. Issues of wealth, status and education, state and religion, and antagonistic knowledges about the body merged here in the *kachinja*-idiom. It was activated by our appearance in the village, but it was used in a long-standing quarrel between two neighbours about land, ideology, and lifestyle. Mr Okoth was thus caught between his wives and the other men, and in response he turned temporarily against his wives and us.

In shifting constellations – researchers versus homestead, second wife and researcher versus younger wives, wives and researcher versus husband, homestead and researcher versus village – *kachinja* was used in different ongoing conflicts involving various overlapping fields of interest. Gradually, our position shifted from being outside the family and a threat to it, to being in some situations a part of it vis-à-vis the rest of the village. At no point had the suspicions lead to a breakdown of contact or violence. The difference established by the idiom was perceived as situational, momentary, tied to changing social relations. After some time, the *kachinja* idiom disappeared from use around us. Blood collection was no longer disputed and people even voluntarily brought children for examinations. The underlying conflicts remained, but if I now mentioned *kachinja*, the topic was no longer met with suspicious silence, but with laughter or accounts of events 'long ago,' 'far away'. The idiom had lost its use-value in the situations at hand and had given way for everyday interactions. It will re-appear, however, once a change in the local situation renders it useful for social practice again.

Conclusion

As its emergence and disappearance in Uhero village shows, *kachinja* is a latent idiom, a narrative that is generally available, but only voiced or realised in practice in a situation of strained relations. It is not a straightforward reflection of specific events, such as research, but it belongs to a store of hypotheses that can be applied to unclear or threatening social situations. Its use depends on whether details of the idiom fit the particular social situation and if significant other persons agree with it, and upon the social or material benefit that its use brings. Neither the conditions nor the social tensions, which render any rumour useful in a given moment, are stable. Thus, rumours are moments, situations in social process. They do not seek out a truth, but question and evaluate experience.

Kachinja is speculative, evaluating, trying out possible understandings and actions. It evokes a possible danger, it does not state facts. It proposes a hypothesis to link empirical facts, memories, and experiences at a specific junction in the social process, and to direct action.

Kachinja is not a permanent social category identifying a person or group as evil blood-thieves, nor is it a defined and bounded political analysis of the capitalist, post-colonial world system. It expresses a temporary relation within it, which changes as part of ongoing social processes. As with all good hypotheses, it is contested and gives way to others, as social life and its evaluation progress, and as people continue their pragmatic search for a way through the uncertainties and concerns of life.

The material presented here shows how colonial and post-colonial tensions are refracted, reflected and transformed on the micro-level of social interaction. Global antagonisms are realised within these fields, in local practices that are shaped by conflicts, for example about gender, generations, land ownership, religion and lifestyle, that are partially independent from the post-colonial condition. Sources of power that partly inhere to these fields (as for example domestic relations) and partly originate outside it (as the state) work on people and influence their social praxis. Tensions within a community are temporarily charged and polarised by wider structural tensions, when encounters like those described here change the existing web of relations. Individual positions, and relations between them, are enforced by powers beyond the confines of the village, when, due to an event like the research-intervention, the *kachinja* idiom is used in social action. Through *kachinja*, global structures of inequality are enacted by local agents, and at the same time global agents (such as the researchers) get entangled into local structures and histories. In their mutual interaction, practices and epistemology of biomedical research are evaluated and criticised in their wider political and economic context. But *kachinja* is more than an 'occult' reflection of the global political economy. Rather, the idiom makes use of historical traditions and lived experiences in order to create a space within which the encounter can be evaluated, and in which global connections are tied into local patterns of relatedness, and both are made to work upon one another.

This example shows how local micro-interactions feed into a framework of local, older ideas and memories. A small spark can ignite them, and small changes in crucial connections can in turn defuse the rumour. A few important people change their attitude, share meals with a researcher, experience mutual support, and the balance tips and nobody talks about the rumour any longer. It remains stored in memory and is reactivated if a pretext arises. In the course of time, what was first a rumour becomes a memory of something that happened, long ago.

Rumours show that in order to devise successful and sustainable medical research and public health interventions we need to be more aware of the context into which local people insert the interventions and the ways in which they talk about them: both the history of a population, and its political and economic situation need to be taken into account, when a project is planned. Rumours, anxieties and misgivings have to be considered when conducting health work. Often, blood sampling and other contentious procedures are critical to the medical work, and these should not be seen as the main problem. What ultimately causes rumours and potentially obstructs public health work is not just what the health workers are doing in medical terms but how they do it in social terms, how relations with community members are established and maintained. If public health workers and researchers do not want to be identified as vampires, these issues will have to be addressed by medical anthropologists in public health.

Summary

In this chapter we introduced science studies and their potential usefulness to medical anthropology in public health. Scientific work neither merely reveals truth or nature, nor is it just a construction by scientists or society. Rather, it is made in concrete practices that connect and disconnect people and things in ever-changing, expansive networks or collectives. If we want to understand scientific knowledge we need to look ethnographically at what scientists and others in scientific research do, and understand their emergent networks. If we in turn want to understand and engage with the knowledge that people other than scientists – such as study populations – produce about research, we should engage them through participant observation with scientific, medical research work. Part of the knowledge produced by science work consists of the stories told among the study populations during and after medical trials. These stories link research interventions to other networks on various levels. On the highest level they link into capitalism or questions of race and inequality; on an intermediate level they link to national history and political processes, and on the micro level to personal and idiosyncratic concerns between people and local groups.

Medical anthropology in public health can contribute to understanding science and communities, and can improve research and health intervention by drawing attention to, revealing and exploring these networks of intentional, unintended and unrecognized connections.

References

Comaroff J and Comaroff JL (1999) Occult economies and the violence of abstraction: notes from the South African postcolony. *American Ethnologist* 26(2): 279–303.

Fairhead J, Leach M and Small M (2004) *Childhood Vaccination and Society in the Gambia: Public Engagement with Science and Delivery*. Brighton: Institute of Development Studies, University of Sussex.

Feldman-Savelsberg P, Ndonko FT and Schmidt-Ehry B (2000) Sterilizing vaccines or the politics of the womb: retrospective study of rumour in Cameroon. *Medical Anthropology Quarterly* 14: 159–79.

Geissler PW (2005) Kachinja are coming: encounters around a medical research project in a Kenyan village. *Africa* 75(2), 173–202.

Hooper E (1999) *The River. A Journey Back to the Source of HIV and AIDS*. Harmondsworth: Penguin.

Latour B (1999) *Pandora's Hope. Essays on the Reality of Science Studies*. Cambridge, Mass.: Harvard University Press.

Molyneux CS, Peshu N and Marsh K (2004) Understanding of informed consent in a low-income setting: three case studies from the Kenyan coast. *Social Science and Medicine* 59(12): 2547–59.

Nchito MF, Geissler PW, Mubila L, Friis H and Olsen A (2003) The effect of iron and multi-micronutrient supplementation on Ascaris lumbricoides reinfection among Zambian schoolchildren – a two by two factorial study. *Transactions of the Royal Society for Tropical Medicine and Hygiene* 98: 218–27.

White L (2000) *Speaking with Vampires: Rumour and History in Colonial Africa*. Berkeley: University of California Press.

Glossary

Aetiology Explanations of the causes of sickness.

Bracketing Setting on hold, or excluding from consideration, certain concepts or aspects of a situation; for example studying a patient's experience of an illness while ignoring (despite being aware of) the biological disease.

Colonial occupation The formal, politically and militarily supported domination and control of territories inhabited by people with another identity, language or culture and a different political constitution, without their consent, with the intent of transforming their societies, cultures, and the aim of benefiting economically (and otherwise) from this.

Commodification Process in which things in people's lives are replaced by commodities, objects that are produced for the purpose of exchange and considered to contain an inherent value that can be translated into the equivalent of another commodity or a monetary exchange medium. Commodification is linked to the replacement of gift economies, in which things derive their value explicitly from social relations, by commodity economies.

Cultural relativism The notion that what is good or right or normal in one society is not necessarily so in another.

Debates An emphasis on debates in ethnographic fieldwork – in contrast to an emphasis on, for example, homogeneous 'local knowledge' – takes into account the fact that no social group is homogeneous, and that it is especially from open debates and confrontations that we can learn about local ideas and practices. Thus we ought to study not 'ideas of' social groups, but 'debates within' them.

Discipline Adapted from the late philosopher Michel Foucault to designate modern forms of social order that apply power to bodies in non-coercive ways. An example of a 'regime of bodily discipline' would be the colonial emphasis on 'hygiene', which transformed domestic and interpersonal practices, reorganized public and private space, and instilled an order of cleanliness and separations that not only reduced disease, but also transported concepts of the person, relations and morality that were part of colonial governance (Fabian 1991: 159–61).

Disease Abnormalities in the structure and function of organs and body systems, as defined by biomedicine.

Dividual Used to capture the observation that, among certain peoples and in particular situations, the person is understood not as individual, but as extending into other persons and things, continuously divided and recomposed through social practices.

Epistemology A branch of philosopy concerned with the nature of knowledge, the different kinds of knowledge that are possible and their limits.

Ethnocentrism The assumption that your own culture, values, ways of doing things – the ones that you have learned and internalized – are the only or the best or the most valid ones.

Ethnography A word with many meanings. 'Ethnography' literally means description of a people or 'ethnic' group. The descriptions that anthropologists write of the people they study are called ethnographies. 'Ethnography' also refers to the actual fieldwork on which anthropologists base their descriptions. Anthropologists *do* ethnography. Sometimes the word is used more broadly to refer to the discipline of anthropology itself.

Ethnomedicine Has been defined as 'those beliefs and practices relating to disease which are the products of indigenous cultural development and are not explicitly derived from the conceptual framework of modern medicine'. In the past, the term referred to the medical systems of 'primitive' or non-Western societies. However, in contemporary medical anthropology biomedicine is not uncritically privileged above other medical systems and biomedicine is also considered to be a form of ethnomedicine.

Explanatory Model (EM) As used by Arthur Kleinman and many of his followers, an explanatory model consists of the ideas about a particular episode of sickness and its treatment that are employed by all those engaged in the clinical process.

Functionalism The theory that society is a unitary whole and that the parts all contribute to the maintenance of the whole. The existence of behaviours or social institutions, and the form they take, are explained in terms of their contribution to the stability of society as a whole.

Generic drugs The basic active component of a pharmaceutical, irrespective of who produced it; in contrast to a 'branded drug', which is the one produced and often patented by a particular company.

Habitus Embodied 'dispositions' that shape and delimit social practice; the concept helps to bridge between 'social structures', 'outside' the person, and 'personal agency' and will, 'inside'. Culture and society are inculcated as a 'habitus' into bodies; persons are constrained as well as enabled by their habitus. For medical anthropology, the habitus is a tool to examine the interrelation of society, body and person in illness and health.

Health belief model A model of health behaviour, very popular in the biomedical and biomedically oriented social science literature, which assumes that behaviour is determined primarily by the 'beliefs' and rational decisions of individuals.

Hegemony The permeation throughout society of a system of values, attitudes, beliefs, and so forth, that supports the status quo and becomes internalized to such an extent that it seems like common sense.

Heuristic Allowing or assisting to discover. In social science, a heuristic device is a model or a concept that, while not necessarily portraying things as they really are, nonetheless helps us to understand them (for example 'culture' or 'medical system').

Illness The patient's subjective experience of physical or mental states, whether based on some underlying disease pathology or not.

Illness narrative Stories that patients (but also friends, relatives, healers) tell about sickness. It is often from these stories, collected during long informal discussions with informants, that anthropologists obtain their information about how people experience sickness and suffering.

Indigenization This term usually applies to the process of adaptation to the local social and cultural environment that Western biomedicine undergoes when it becomes part of non-Western medical systems. However, it could also refer to the inclusion of aspects of non-Western medical traditions into biomedicine (for example acupuncture).

Individual Used here in the sense of a construct of the person that stresses autonomy, separateness, independence.

Kwashiorkor A severe form of protein-energy malnutrition.

Materialism The theory that everything that really exists is material, and that mental states or consciousness are merely derived from material substance.

Medical pluralism The existence, within one medical system, or one society, of different medical traditions.

Medicalization The extension of biomedicine into areas of life that previously were considered social rather than medical (for example, birth and dying), and the expansion of the power and influence of medical experts, sometimes even to the extent that medicine takes on a deviance control function (for instance, in child-abuse cases).

Medicine Substances (or objects) that, based on their inherent potency, are employed to engender transformations, such as the bodily change from ill health to health.

Modern A concept that order the world by opposing itself to what belongs to the past: tradition. A narrative device that organizes time, space and social differences around the fiction of a great leap forward in history – the gap between those who made the leap and those who did not (yet) do so and remain 'traditional'.

Mystification A process by which the nature of reality is hidden in such a way that it serves to maintain the status quo and protect those in power from criticism.

Network Different from 'social groups', 'networks' are potentially open ended and not defined by boundaries or a core and can be extended and changed continuously. The term emphasizes the connections between different nodes, and the possibility of multiple connections of each node, rather than the essential identity of the 'group' or the individual member of the group. What counts is what links actors, not what they are by themselves.

Occult Used to designate explanations of social practice that refer to secret or unheard-of forces. It would earlier have been called 'magic', but this is now avoided because it connotes stereotypes such as that of 'African witchcraft'. The concept allows exploration of similarities between 'occult' ideas in, for example, the United States (such as the idea that extraterrestrial aliens have assumed power in the White House) and in Africa (such as rumours about blood-selling politicians). It perpetuates the notion of fundamentally different knowledges – 'magical' or 'occult', and 'scientific' or 'rational' – and cannot be a valid analytical term, but is a temporary label for an interesting field of anthropological inquiry.

Pharmaceutical Medicine that is based on biomedical knowledge and industrially produced.

Popularization When aspects of a professional medical tradition (usually biomedicine) filter down into the popular sector (for example, the informal sale of antibiotics, back street injectionists). It could also refer to the popular use of aspects of other medical traditions (for example, the sale of Ayurvedic teas and remedies in British supermarkets).

Positivism The view that there is a reality that exists outside and independently of the observer and that can be directly apprehended. That the scientific method is the only way of obtaining accurate information on this reality, and that value judgements and subjective experiences cannot be a valid basis for knowledge.

Possession States in which persons are displaced, subdued or struggling with spirits, who temporarily determine the body's actions, including speech.

Postcolonial A qualification of periods, societies, nations or ideas after formal colonial occupation; sometimes used as impartial temporal definition, but more commonly to draw attention to the lasting impact of the colonial period.

Reductionism The notion that complex phenomena can be explained by reducing them to some more basic level; for example the idea that disease is basically the physical malfunctioning of organs and cells.

Reification When an abstraction that we have created to help us to understand reality (for example, a concept or a model) is seen as something concrete, that really exists and exerts a causal influence (for instance, culture causes risk behaviour).

Resistance Practices that challenge the exercise of domination through overt struggle or insidious forms of resilience (work-evasion, sabotage, religious activity, drinking, or even sickness).

Risk Risk is a term with many diverse but inter-related meanings. According to the *Oxford English Dictionary*, 'risk' is the chance of danger, loss, injury or other adverse consequences. This resembles the popular use of the term. In epidemiology 'risk' refers to the statistical probability of a particular outcome. For example when marriage is described as a risk factor for HIV infection in Africa, it means that statistically women who are married have higher rates of infection than those who are single. This usage has led to the idea of 'risk behaviours', which has in turn led to the identification (and sometimes stigmatization) of risk groups. This problematic aspect of the concept of risk is discussed in detail in the readings below.

Rumour Narratives, often orally distributed, that serve as a means to discuss experiences; reaching beyond the facts that are generally agreed on about these experiences, or combining known features in innovative ways. The power of rumours to make people act lies in the fact that they are not bound to agreed facts, one can believe in them and doubt them at the same time, and they can be neither proven nor falsified. Therefore, they can suddenly gain mobilizing force in a particular situation, and equally quickly dissolve and vanish from public debate and become 'just a story' again.

Sickness Some medical anthropologists use the term 'sickness' as a cover term to refer to both illness and disease. Others give 'sickness' a more specialized meaning, using it to refer to the process in which illness and disease are socialized. Here we use the term in the former sense, unless specified.

(Social) constructivism This approach to knowledge denies the existence of reality prior to human engagement and the validity of 'truth' in the sense of a corresponding representation of reality. Instead, it poses that reality is whatever is known, and that all knowledge is socially produced. Constructivism can thus lead to relativism, as it allows no distinction between true and untrue statements.

Sociality The practices that the people engage in to establish, maintain or dissolve, emphasize or hide, social relationships (different from 'society', which implies a bounded whole, constituted by an assembly of individual units that enter into relations).

Structural violence The constraints on behaviour and options imposed by institutionalized inequalities in wealth and power on those who are underprivileged: mainly women, the poor, those of colour.

Syncretism A term taken from relgious studies, refers to unifying or reconciling different or opposing schools of thought.

Traditional Used in opposition to 'modern', with connotations of local (versus global or universal), static (versus dynamic), of the past (versus of today and the future). There is no 'tradition' without 'modernity', and vice versa as both concepts are mutually constituted.

Index

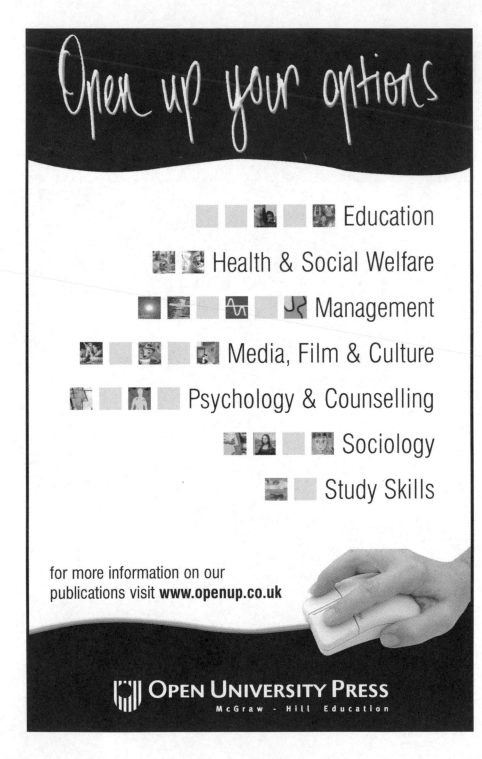